Shaping Global Health Policy

Shaping Global Health Policy

Global Social Policy Actors and Ideas about Health Care Systems

Alexandra Kaasch

Bielefeld University, Germany

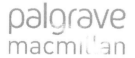

First published 2015 by
PALGRAVE MACMILLAN

Palgrave Macmillan in the UK is an imprint of Macmillan Publishers Limited, registered in England, company number 785998, of Houndmills, Basingstoke, Hampshire RG21 6XS.

Palgrave Macmillan in the US is a division of St Martin's Press LLC, 175 Fifth Avenue, New York, NY 10010.

Palgrave Macmillan is the global academic imprint of the above companies and has companies and representatives throughout the world.

Palgrave® and Macmillan® are registered trademarks in the United States, the United Kingdom, Europe and other countries.

ISBN 978–1–137–30888–7

This book is printed on paper suitable for recycling and made from fully managed and sustained forest sources. Logging, pulping and manufacturing processes are expected to conform to the environmental regulations of the country of origin.

A catalogue record for this book is available from the British Library.

A catalog record for this book is available from the Library of Congress.

To Imke, Gitte and Bernhard

Contents

Acknowledgements

This book was written during the turbulent times of a junior researcher fighting to achieve the dream of "getting in". In my first year of studies at the Free University of Berlin, my favourite professor, Gesine Schwan, asked me about my future plans. I told her I would like to work in academia. She encouraged me but also said "it is a very hard road". Luckily, in one's early twenties, it is easy to believe "I am strong enough". Later on, I often thought about what she'd said, and it helped to know that somebody like Gesine Schwan, a role model in many ways, did not suggest it was easy.

Now, looking back at some of the stages of this "hard road", this book is finally published. This would have never happened without Bob Deacon's constant support and encouragement. Thank you so much, for everything! I discussed my work with many colleagues over the years; there isn't space to mention all of them here. Special thanks to Lutz Leisering, Rianne Mahon, Kerstin Martens, Paul Stubbs and Rebecca Surender for encouragement and "mentoring". Thanks also to Meri Koivusalo, Veronika Wodsak, Jo Ingold, Amy Barnes and Claus Wendt for comments on my work. Katharina and Derya provided editorial help in the final stages of writing. Thanks to Dominic Walker and colleagues from Palgrave Macmillan for being endlessly patient.

I am deeply indebted to Imke, who has supported me in every possible way, and to my children Marieke, Joshua and Sophie. I would also like to thank my parents, Gitte and Bernhard, for "giving the horse the legs to run". Thanks to all of you, as well as Margarete, Hans, Mocki, Hilde, Siegfried and a number of babysitters and au-pairs who made it possible for me to enjoy working and travelling even when the children fell ill and we were lacking childcare. My brother Andreas was always there when the computer went on strike.

Abbreviations and Acronyms

BCA	Biennial collaborative agreement
BRICS	Brazil, Russia, India, China, South Africa
CCM	Country Coordination Mechanism
CEAS	Centre de estudios y asesoria en salud
CMH	Commission on Macroeconomics and Health (WHO)
CRC	Convention on the Rights of the Child
CSDH	Commission on the Social Determinants of Health (WHO)
CSO	Civil society organisation
DAC	Development Assistance Committee (OECD)
DAH	Development assistance for health
DALY	Disability-adjusted life year
DELSA	Directorate for Employment, Labour and Social Affairs (OECD)
EB	Executive Board (WHO)
ECOSOC	Economic and Social Council (UN)
EDRC	Economic Development Review Committee (OECD)
EU	European Union
GA	General Assembly (UN)
GASPP	Globalism and Social Policy Programme
GATS	General Agreement on Trade in Services (WTO)
GAVI	Global Alliance for Vaccines and Immunization
GDN	Global Development Network
GEGA	Global Equity Gauge Alliance
GTZ	German Enterprise for Technical Cooperation
HEG	G8 Health Experts' Group
HFA	Health for All
HIA	Health Impact Assessment
HiT	Health systems in transition
HMO	Health Maintenance Organisations
HNP	Health, Nutrition and Population (World Bank)
IBRD	International Bank for Reconstruction and Development
ICCPR	International Covenant on Civil and Political Rights
ICESCR	International Covenant on Economic, Social and Cultural Rights

IDA	International Development Association
IDPF	International Drug Purchasing Facility
IFC	International Finance Corporation (World Bank Group)
IFFIm	International Finance Facility for Immunisation
IFI	International Financial Institution
IHP	International Health Partnership
ILC	International Labour Conference (ILO)
ILO	International Labour Organization
IMF	International Monetary Fund
INGO	International non-governmental organisation
IPCC	Intergovernmental Panel on Climate Change
ISSA	International Social Security Association
KRUS	Agricultural Social Insurance Fund (Poland)
LIC	Low-income country
MDG	Millennium Development Goal
MIC	Middle-income country
NAM	Non-Aligned Movement
NFZ	National Health Fund (Poland)
NGO	Non-governmental organisation
ODA	Official Development Assistance
OECD	Organisation for Economic Co-operation and Development
OEEC	Organisation for European Economic Co-operation
OWG	Open Working Group for Sustainable Development Goals
PHC	Primary health care
PHI	Private Health Insurance
PHM	People's Health Movement
SDGs	Sustainable Development Goals
STD	Sexually transmitted disease
STEP	Strategies and Tools against social Exclusion and Poverty (ILO)
SWEF	Systemwide Effects of the Fund
TRIPS	Trade-Related Aspects of Intellectual Property Rights (WTO)
UHC	Universal health coverage
UN	United Nations
UNAIDS	United Nations Programme on HIV/AIDS
UNDP	United Nations Development Programme

UNFPA	United Nations Population Fund
UNICEF	United Nations Children's Fund
WEF	World Economic Forum
WHA	World Health Assembly (WHO)
WHO	World Health Organization
WSF	World Social Forum
WTO	World Trade Organization
ZUS	Zakład Ubezpieczeń Społecznych (Polish Social Insurance Institution)

1
Global Social Policy Actors and Health Care System Ideas

1.1 Introduction

Health is a significant global issue, and has become even more so in the past few decades owing to manifold globalisation processes. People all over the world struggle with similar health constraints. The search for curative and eradicative means to cure diseases is usually considered a common and global human challenge. Infectious diseases threaten people in a world of extensive worldwide cross-border exchanges. The dramatic social risks of the inability to work for health reasons affect the lives of people, without regard for age, social status or their place of residence. At the same time, the increasing transnationalisation of family structures and individual work and employment histories poses significant challenges to national and supranational health care provision and financing.

An important institution to tackle such challenges is the health care system (also referred to as "health system").[1] While commonly set up at national policy levels, health care systems as concepts or strategies also form a central element of global social policy agendas and debates. They are considered important for the achievement of global health goals (such as the health-related Millennium Development Goals (MDGs) and the post-2015 goals (so-called Sustainable Development Goals (SDGs)), and they provide a key element of various other social development and global health strategies; for example, when it concerns the fight against specific diseases. In a speech to the United Nations (UN) General Assembly meeting on the

Prevention and Control of Non-Communicable Diseases (2011), UN Secretary-General Ban Ki-moon stated:

> Improving health systems improves health services. Involving all parts of government attacks all sides of a problem. And taking comprehensive action is the best way to protect against diseases.

The vital importance of well-functioning health care systems appears to be common knowledge among national and global policymakers, and a vital goal in high-, middle- and low-income countries alike. Nevertheless, the great challenges and considerable uncertainties with regard to building up, and maintaining, functioning health care systems seem to be equally shared in national and transnational policy arenas. One can find political efforts in various places, and at different levels of policymaking, to address issues such as long-term sustainable funding of health care systems, equal and adequate health provision and access to health care. At the same time demographic changes, technical innovation and different forms of crisis (such as global economic crises, disease outbreaks and natural catastrophes) create stresses on national health care systems.

In such situations, on the one hand, "health care systems" as a global health topic appear to be particularly important, and national and global actors alike call for increased attention on more comprehensive – or horizontal – approaches to health care systems that go beyond tackling specific diseases (so-called vertical approaches). On the other hand, however, the complexity and relative costs of health care systems frequently appear insurmountable. That often results in new initiatives to tackle specific problems in the short term, and just *talking* about the need to focus on health care systems more generally.

1.2   Global health policy and governance

The unquestionable importance of health care systems for the well-being of individual societies, together with the marked lack of straightforward solutions to major questions of health and social protection, has generated multi-scaled, transnational activities concerning national health care systems. The related initiatives partly connect to specific health issues (such as the fight against malaria or tuberculosis). Partly, however, they also reflect global ideational discourse as a somewhat independent sphere of global social and health policy. Some of these discourses relate to particular groups of countries or regions; while others are supposed to apply in general and globally.

More generally, global governance of health care systems, or global health governance, is characterised by a typical multi-layered, polyarchic and pluralistic institutional architecture. We can observe a variable geometry in the sense of varying political significance and regulatory capacities in different parts of the world, or by different actors (on global social governance more specifically, see Kaasch and Martens, 2015). This architecture is, in addition, in a process of continuous change; and ever new configurations of actors, as well as a continuously growing number of different kinds of actors, activities, overlapping jurisdictions, power resources and competencies result in a growing complexity (Held and McGrew, 2002: 5; Wilkinson, 2002: 2; Hein and Kohlmorgen, 2008).

Accordingly, we find a great number and variety of transnational policy actors dedicating (part of) their attention and resources to the topic of health care systems. "Health care systems" have found their way into the world's major international meetings, such as the World Economic Forum and G20 Summits. International (governmental) organisations such as the World Health Organization (WHO) and the World Bank commit substantial resources to analyse and support health care systems in various ways. Numerous civil society organisations (CSOs), including philanthropic organisations, provide significant support to health care systems by advocacy, donations and direct provision of health care. In their exchange of ideas, their interrelatedness and their collaborations, these global social and health policy actors represent a global sphere, or level, of policymaking on the issue of health care systems.

This book is concerned with questions such as: What do global actors do in order to guide national health care systems? What are their ideas? How do these ideas compare? And how can they be related to national health policies?

1.3   Global health policy as global social policy

The literature on global social policy and governance (for example, Deacon et al., 1997; Yeates, 2001, 2008; Orenstein, 2005, 2008; Deacon, 2007; Kaasch and Stubbs, 2014; Kaasch and Martens, 2015) and global health governance (for example, Lee et al., 2002; Hein and Kohlmorgen, 2003, 2008; Lee, 2003; Kickbusch, 2004) have revealed, illustrated and explained many of the characteristics just described. This book intends to contribute to the global social policy literature in reporting a detailed study in a social policy field that has been rather neglected within the past years, namely health care systems. It draws on the insights provided in that literature, but it also challenges and updates some of the information and accounts. Apart from Koivusalo and Ollila (1997), the existing contributions have either focused on global social policy, or social policy and globalisation more generally, or primarily on the field of pensions (for example, Müller, 2003; Brooks, 2005, 2007; Ervik, 2005; Orenstein, 2005, 2008, 2011; Weyland, 2005). Other contributions are rather organisation-driven, and study the role of the World Bank (for example, St Clair, 2006), the WHO (for example, Siddiqi, 1995; Lee, 2009) or the Organisation for Economic Co-operation and Development (OECD) (for example, Mahon and McBride, 2008b; Martens and Jakobi, 2010). By drawing on a broad picture of various global social policy actors, this book follows the approach used to study international actors and their social policy ideas as developed and employed by Bob Deacon, but with a focus on a particular social policy field (for example, Deacon et al., 1997). Such a contribution will enable us to better understand some of the nuances of global social policy discourses and struggles over positions, going beyond a general take on the issue that merely offers broad and general accounts of global social policy, without considering the potential differences between social policy fields.

The issues and discussions addressed in this book are conceptualised as a form of global social policy and governance. Health care systems as an issue of global policies and governance matter in different ways. Following Deacon's (2007) understanding of global social policy, a distinction can be made between "truly" or genuinely global social policies, and prescriptions for national social policy generated and disseminated by global social policy actors. The dimension of a genuinely global social policy involves mechanisms of global social redistribution, the formulation of global social rights and the enactment of global social regulation. Theoretically, related to health care systems, this could add up to something approaching a "global health care system". Indeed, global social redistribution happens predominantly through the field of health. Many of the innovative financing facilities are connected to health issues (such as the International Finance Facility for Immunisation (IFFIm), or the International Drug Purchasing Facility (IDPF)). There are further global funds for supporting health development, most importantly the Global Fund to Fight Aids, Tuberculosis, and Malaria (Global Fund) (discussed in Chapter 5). In terms of international organisations, there is, for example, the ILO Ghana-Luxembourg Social Trust project scheme (2009–2014) that provided families in Ghana with health care coverage through subsidisation of their premiums.[2] Apart from the funding to fight particular diseases and/or supporting health care systems, such organisations, initiatives and programmes also carry particular ideas about health care systems and in that way influence national health policy reforms. Another issue within this global social policy dimension is connected to the definition and potential provision of global public goods (Kaul et al., 1999, 2003). Health plays an important role, as a number of health issues have been identified as having a "global public good" character, such as the global surveillance of infectious diseases (as through the WHO) or the global control of tobacco consumption and illicit drugs (the WHO's Framework Convention on Tobacco Control is an important document in this context (Jha and Chaloupka, 2000; WHO, 2005 (updated reprint); see also, for example, Gilmore et al., 2007).

Concerning global social regulation, critical issues are international or global labour and social standards, trade matters, voluntary codes of conduct by business, global tax regulation and migration. In contrast to the dimension of redistribution where health issues are a key field of activity, this is less so for regulation. However, an important discussion in this context is that of the implications of trade agreements and the World Trade Organization's (WTO) role in the health sector. The concern here is that through facilitating trade also in social and health services, detrimental effects on the health of people and social security systems can arise (for example, Koivusalo, 1999, 2003a, 2003b, 2003c; Pollock and Price, 2000; Sexton, 2001; Holden, 2003, 2005) (for a related discussion see Chapter 3). Another issue, connected to migration and particularly relevant to health, is "brain drain", which refers to the weakening of health care systems through staff shortages caused by migration (for example, Martineau et al.,

2004; Kapur and McHale, 2005). Further, global food standards are also related to health issues (see for example Post, 2005).

As the third element of a global social policy, global social rights have to be considered. These represent a particular type of rights as – compared to civil and political rights – they require resources in order to be met (Deacon, 2007: 136; Kaasch, forthcoming). Such social rights have been formulated, amongst others, in the International Covenant on Economic, Social and Cultural Rights (ICESCR) of 1976, the Universal Declaration of Human Rights of 1948, the Convention on the Rights of the Child (CRC) of 1990 and the International Covenant on Civil and Political Rights (ICCPR) of 1976. Rights issues are particularly important in the context of gender, ethnicity or other issues that are prone to discriminatory practices; and include health-related rights (see for example Mishra, 1999; Deacon, 2007; Tarantola, 2008). Tarantola shows how health as a social right came into focus in the context of dealing with HIV/AIDS, because of the belief that "human rights were [...] a prerequisite for open access to prevention and care by those who needed them most; away from fear, discrimination and other forms of human rights violations" (Tarantola, 2008: 15). On a similar topic, Hein and Kohlmorgen (2008) engage with new institutional structures in global health governance with a focus on HIV/AIDS and global social rights. These issues are also important for the organisation of health care systems.

Even when taking all these forms of a truly global social policy that relate to health policies and health care systems together, we are far from a truly global health care system. These forms of global social and health policy are only examples of what is happening at the global level with regard to health. Particularly regarding the second form of global social policy as supranational social policy, this is also connected to a potential future global welfare state, as discussed by Leisering (2007), or a global health care system, as envisaged by Kickbusch (2003).

From a normative perspective, despite valid claims about reducing global inequalities on health, it might still not be desirable or feasible to work towards such an institution, given great differences in health needs and cultural expectations.

Turning to the global prescriptions for health care systems, numerous global health actors provide information and recommendations in the form of models and suggestions for reforms of health care systems. As such, prescriptions are only comprehensive in some cases; they are seldom complete and coherent. This often makes it complicated to capture and characterise them. Different perspectives on national health care systems play a role, as well as the different contexts within which health care systems are being addressed by specific actors. However, it needs to be taken into account that the discussion in this book about global actors in health care system issues is less about empirical, national health care systems and experiences, but mainly concerns global ideas and models (with the exception of Chapter 7, which makes the move towards implications for national health care systems, namely Poland).

1.4   Approaches to study global prescriptions for health care systems

Analytically and methodologically, the following approaches have been employed to understand global social policy actors and ideas, and their application at the national policy level. Studies of policy diffusion and transfer in general, as well as case studies for specific (groups of) countries or policy fields have shown that national social and health policy is being influenced by external factors; and these studies have analysed such processes between states as they relate to national policymaking in a single country. Usually, diffusion studies include, amongst other things, findings that relate to policy change through the creation and spread of new ideas; and geographical clustering. They look at the "spread of commonality amid diversity", and often concentrate on mechanisms of diffusion (Orenstein, 2003; Meseguer, 2004). Interdependence of decisions taken in different places is an important characteristic of diffusion processes (Braun and Gilardi, 2006). Elkins and Simmons (2005: 39) define this interdependence as uncoordinated; thus, "the actions and choices of one country affect another but not through any collaboration, imposition or otherwise programmed effort on the part of any of the actors".

Also policy transfer analyses focus on external influences on national policy, though with a different approach. The basic assumption is that policymakers are increasingly looking at what is going on in other places, and thus, according to Dolowitz and Marsh (2000), the implementation of new policies includes an iterative process of policy transfer between different contexts. They define policy transfer as the process of bringing ideas, programmes, institutions, policies, administrative arrangements and so on from one place and/or time into another place and/or time (Dolowitz and Marsh, 2000).

While transfer and diffusion studies provide evidence and examples of national social policy being influenced by external factors, the emphasis on processes between societal units often neglects the importance of the – sometimes quite concrete – localities and instances of supranational policy actors. The role of international organisations in influencing national social policy has been emphasised by the literature on global social policy employing international actors approaches (for example, Deacon, 2007; Orenstein, 2008), analysing the activities and power of international organisations (and other actors at that policy level). This includes studying the content of policy advice given by international organisations and other actors, as well as their strategies or activities in disseminating those ideas at global level and towards nation states (Deacon et al., 1997).

In this book, the approach employed focuses on three analytical units to understand the global actors that are engaged in providing prescriptions for health systems. These are mandates, ideas and dissemination mechanisms. The following sections describe the meaning and use of these categories.

1.5   Organisations and mandates

Global health policy and governance in the form of ideas about, and prescriptions for, national health care systems sets the stage for quite a number of international governmental and non-governmental organisations that are developing and disseminating knowledge or ideas about the structure, performance and reform of health care systems. They do this, however, with different mandates, and some of these activities are an expression of a system of global governance that is not characterised by a clear division of labour, but by parallel processes resulting in overlapping and to some extent competing agencies (Deacon, 2007; Kaasch, 2007). That means that a number of international organisations and other actors have identified health care systems as an issue relevant to achieving their particular aims, be they supporting a particular group of people (such as the United Nations Children's Fund (UNICEF) for children), tackling a specific problem or achieving broader development aims (such as the United Nations Development Programme (UNDP) or the World Bank).

Instead of discussing and questioning different global health actors from a normative perspective, concerning the ways in which they use their power and disseminate particular ideas, this book considers the type of involvement by a particular organisation on the basis of the mandate given to it, or the expressed purpose for its engagement. This allows us to understand the justification of a particular actor's involvement in the topic area, and provides the basis for comparing involvement and ideas. Basically, following Orenstein (2005: 177), "global policy actors are defined by the scope of their policy activity, not their constitutional nature". In order to contextualise this involvement and give appropriate justice to the scope or content of the ideas developed and disseminated, it is nevertheless crucial to understand their mandates when analysing their activities, but even more so when making claims about the justification of a particular organisation's involvement in a specific policy issue. Such "mandates", however, naturally take very different forms for different types of actor. In the global health literature, Koivusalo and Ollila (1997) have employed the approach to systematically trace global health organisations' mandates.

1.6 Concepts and ideas

In order to illustrate the key actors in global social policies around health care systems, and to describe and compare their respective ideas and relationships, health care systems are conceptualised with regard to their functions as being parts of broader systems of social protection (welfare states). This includes the definitions and functions of health care systems, such as the provision of health services, and the financing and regulation of health care systems (conceptually related to the work of Rothgang and his research group, Rothgang et al., 2005, 2010). These concepts and distinctions are applied in the analysis reported in this book, and are different from other conceptual distinctions; for example, the distinction between so-called comprehensive Primary Health Care (PHC) approaches, usually connected with WHO and other UN social agencies (see Chapter 2), and those of selective health approaches, associated with UNICEF and the international financial institutions (IFIs) (see for example Koivusalo and Ollila, 1997). Also different is the common distinction between vertical approaches (that are, in their "pure" form, programmes or interventions that concentrate on a single disease and are usually organised independently) and horizontal approaches (encompassing several health interventions within a more comprehensive primary care approach) (see for example Victora et al., 2004). While this book addresses and includes horizontal and vertical approaches in its analysis, it does not use this terminology and these concepts in terms of its analytical approach. Health care systems as global social policy ideas cannot be fully equated with horizontal approaches – rather, we can say that periods of interest in horizontal approaches have provided a platform for engaging more thoroughly with health care systems.

In a national context, what is referred to as a health care system is different depending on the discipline and perspective within which the topic is being addressed. To only mention a few, health economics is primarily interested in studying the financing of health care provision or services. It is also concerned about how to improve the health status of the population, while maintaining fairness or equity between the members of a society, and defending the view that choices have to be made between the different goals pursued through health care systems. Sociological perspectives tend to regard health care systems as specialised subsystems of society, with the totality of health care systems in a society adding up to one (national) health care system, and existing next to other functionally relevant systems such as education. Accordingly, a health care system is defined as the "social mechanism that has arisen or been devised to deal with the incapacitating aspects of illness, trauma and (to some degree) premature mortality" (Field, 1973: 765). Public health studies, originating from medical, sociological or anthropological perspectives, typically focus on the health of particular groups of the population and make assumptions about the improvement of the health of the population (such as smoking or tobacco control), but the interest extends to health care system issues. Gill Walt (1994: 41), for example, defined health policy as "embrac[ing] courses of action that affect the set of institutions, organisations, services, and funding arrangements for the health care system". However, health policy is often also linked to the concept of "public policy that aims to explain the interaction between institutions, interests and ideas in the policy process" (Walt et al., 2008: 308). A common feature of such studies is also that health policy is directly linked to health outcomes. A health care system approach as employed by Mackintosh and Koivusalo (2005) tries to combine the economic approach to health care systems with one of public health and medical systems. They define, therefore, "health policies and health care systems [...] [as] public policies and health policies [that] form part of the broader public policy framework in a society", and point to the fact that health policies "are also part of normative policy-making within a society, and embedded in legal rights and commitments made as part of public policies" (Mackintosh and Koivusalo, 2005: 5). Last but not least, social policy or welfare state studies regard health care systems as one element of a broader welfare state, facilitating social security for the citizens or inhabitants of a nation state. The models, or regime types, of health care systems, derived from comparative welfare state analysis, attempt to identify specific types of welfare state arrangements for handling the consequences of illness and treatment.

We do not only find such different perspectives with regard to different academic disciplines and fields. They are also present in global discourses, where in the sense of discourses taking place within and between international organisations acting as global social policy actors, the use of the term health (care) systems is far from coherent. There are important differences in the underlying goals and principles with which health care systems are being approached by different global actors. Not only different organisations, but also different documents by one organisation may express different perspectives and assumptions in approaching health care systems. Of course, those might not be entirely mutually exclusive, and many documents enumerate a number of goals or principles which may be partly overlapping. However, the documents (the entire approach taken by one particular organisation) are usually driven by a single conception of what a health care system is, what the most relevant issues are and which options are worth considering when thinking about health care reform.

1.7   Dissemination mechanisms

There are several different sources or mechanisms that global social and health policy actors use to influence national policymaking. One might think of legal means (for example, European law, international labour standards deriving from the ILO or health regulation facilitated by the WHO), financial power (usually discussed in the literature on the World Bank and its loans) or external pressures in the form of obligations on states by means of economic integration – a rather indirect, though certainly not less powerful form (for example, the European Union (EU)). The potential power of most global health actors lies in producing and disseminating ideas, namely defining problems and providing solutions, proposing policy or reform models and so on; and diffusing or transferring such ideas to the national policymaking level. McNeill (2005: 58) defines such ideas as "collective images" that influence policy and develop through the "interplay between the academic and policy domains" – in the context of this analysis the focus is on the knowledge produced in international organisations that colludes with national policy domains. In this form of "ideational" influence, the more developed European countries are not necessarily less receptive than less developed countries, which are usually considered to be more exposed to external actors' influence on their national policies.

Global policy actors may have a number of different functions and use different strategies/channels when it comes to providing models for national policy. Deacon (2007: 24) lists research, agenda setting and the development of knowledge frameworks; policy-based lending and project conditionality; and establishing global codes, rules and norms. Similarly, Stone and Maxwell (2005) stress the roles of being sources of normative standards; as research institutions producing and communicating knowledge about social policy issues. They can further provide "meeting points" for national governments for policy exchange and mutual learning. The potential power of the ideas-related mechanisms may unfold through the link with redistributive or regulatory functions and influences, such as through the use of aid connected with conditionalities.

While often rather employing quantitative methods, approaches to studying policy diffusion (Meyer et al., 1997) provide important insights into the spread of universal knowledge. Most diffusion definitions focus on the level of process, rather than the result or outcome of diffusion (Elkins and Simmons, 2005). Leisering (2005: 78) remarks that it is important to distinguish between the two, but taking into account that there is more than process. While this is not the place to discuss all characteristics of diffusion in detail, the mechanisms of diffusion are important in this context (Orenstein, 2003; Braun and Gilardi, 2005). A number of such diffusion mechanisms can be identified (Elkins and Simmons, 2004) and they vary slightly from one author to another. Braun and Gilardi (2005: 12ff.), for example, distinguish between learning, competitive interdependence, cooperative interdependence, coercion, common norms, taken-for-granted and symbolic imitation.

Orenstein (2003: 174) defines the categories for diffusion mechanisms as interstate competition for economic resources and legitimacy, the role of interstate organisations, the role of epistemic communities in spreading new ideas and information about policy reform, and the role of regional models in demonstrating policy feasibility. Elkins and Simmons (2005: 4) distinguish between "those [diffusion mechanisms] for which another's adoption alters the value of the practice and those for which another's adoption imparts information". For the first category, adoption to altered conditions, they further distinguish between cultural norms, support groups and competition. For the second one, learning, they identify different methods, namely information cascades, learning and availability, and learning and reference groups.

Similar is the policy transfer approach, conceptually developed by Dolowitz and Marsh (2000). Policy transfer is described as the process of bringing ideas, programmes, institutions, policies or administrative arrangements from one place and/or time into another place and/or time. This process can take different shapes, such as lesson drawing, coercive policy transfer, policy harmonisation or cross-national policy learning. The basic assumptions of the policy transfer approach are that, owing to global economic forces and the growth of communications of all types, the exchange of information is growing. International organisations are one type of facilitator of influence on national policies (Dolowitz and Marsh, 2000: 5ff.).

Formal negotiations usually take place in the context of international conferences, such as meetings of official representatives of member states to a particular organisation, or of a particular group in society. Such gatherings may lead to forms of international health regulation or provide forums for policy learning. They are also an important opportunity for the organising party, for example international organisations secretariats' staff or people working for a global think tank, to foster particular ideas about an issue through agenda-setting and the distribution of background material. This, then, links with the second important mechanism of spreading ideas, namely various forms of publications, such as strategy papers, advocacy reports and research documents. In particular, advocacy documents can serve as important means to inform the international community and shape the perception of global health problems and their possible solutions, while research documents can be influential in shaping the understanding of how to define and measure a national or global health problem, and by that way also the possible scope of solutions. Mutual learning can also be facilitated at conferences and workshops organised by international organisations and other actors. These are used to inform and "teach" national policymakers and/or staff from other organisations. Such events also use publications by the organising organisation and others, and also academic publications, as background material, as they often invite the exchange of national policymakers and/or bureaucrats related to specific policy or reform issues. More direct involvement in national policymaking may happen through financial (conditional) support and project activity, often combined with advice about the structure and reform of policies. Global health policy actors may further engage in developing indicators, and collecting and reporting data. This also sometimes includes the ranking of countries, or lengthy reports of a country's performance in a particular policy field. The websites and connected means (such as email lists and newsletters) are of course also part of an organisation's communication channels. They present the respective organisations and spread information and knowledge. Related to particular sets of ideas are also campaigns to advocate a particular policy model or idea. Finally, global policy actors build up and participate in networks or epistemic communities that also lead to a spread of ideas, to the promotion of particular models, and the definition and common use of terminology.

1.8   Inter-actor relationships

In terms of the structures of global governance involved in the field of global policy prescriptions for national health care systems, a number of points stand out. As mentioned before, global health governance involves numerous actors, including international governmental organisations, international non-governmental organisations (INGOs), other actors, legal frameworks, public-private partnerships, national programmes and so on that make up the complicated governance structure in health policies and their cross-border dimensions (see for example Musgrove, 1999; Thomas and Weber, 2004; Hein and Kohlmorgen, 2008). The scene has been most usefully mapped by Koivusalo and Ollila (1997) and by Lee and Goodman (2002), particularly regarding health financing more specifically. Under the term 'global health governance', there has been a whole range of further studies focusing on related issues (for example, Dodgson and Lee, 2002; Hein and Kohlmorgen, 2003; Cooper et al., 2007). The role, and ambiguous power, of the WHO in particular has been addressed for example by Peabody (1995), Siddiqi (1995) and Taylor (2002). The World Bank's health activities are the focus of contributions from Ruger (2005) and Beyer et al. (2000); and recently the International Finance Corporation (IFC) also gained attention as an emerging actor in global health (see Wogart, 2003; Lethbridge, 2005) (Chapter 2 deals with these actors). Important to mention here is also the WTO, which is increasingly emerging as a global health actor, as demonstrated and discussed for example in the work by Koivusalo (1999, 2003b) and Holden (2005) (in this book addressed in Chapter 3). Further, and particularly important for the health field, is the work of philanthropic foundations, public-private partnerships (Buse and Walt, 2000, 2002; Bartsch, 2003, 2007) and the role of the hybrid organisation of the Global Fund (for example, Bartsch, 2005) (see Chapter 5).

We also have to consider the diverse linkages between actors, such as collaborations between, or transnational networks of, such actors (Deacon et al., 1997). Deacon found there is a

> shift in the locus and content of policy debate and activity [...] to a set of practices around Networks, Partnerships and Projects which, in some way bypass, the [...] [more formal] institutions and debate and present new possibilities for actually making global change in particular policy arenas.
>
> (2003: 27)

This suggests two things: on the one hand, global policy actors do not operate in isolation; but on the other hand, we do not have a global government with clearly ascribed roles and responsibilities at a supranational level. Such discussions about the functions and organisations, but also about the general structures of governance at transnational policy levels, have been discussed under the heading of global social or health governance (see also Deacon, 2007; Kaasch and Martens, 2015).

International organisations and other organisations are sometimes regarded as generally "good" actors. They usually try to sell their work as "impersonal, technocratic, and neutral – as not exercising power but instead as serving others" (Barnett and Finnemore, 1999: 708). Other authors, however, have been concerned and very critical about particular international organisations' (potential) power and content of activities (for example, Kapur, 1998). More specifically, Vaughan (1999) looks at the "dark side of organizations" and analyses different forms of shortcomings in her work. There is also a tendency of "mission creep" and expansion of original mandates (Einhorn, 2001) that might result in unintended consequences. Similar concerns regarding the generally positive intention and role exist towards CSO and philanthropic engagement, accompanied by a parallel concern about unintended consequences and inadequate representation through the work of these actors.

The way that international organisations and other actors have just been described suggests they function as actors to some degree independently of their member states or other kinds of members (NGOs, individuals). However, apart from the question of the dependence or independence from their member states or other composing units, these organisations also often collaborate on particular topics or issue areas. When they build alliances, these are often referred to, and studied as, networks. In contrast to understandings of networks as a modern form of policy process (Castells, 2000; Keohane and Nye, 2000) or as a means for transfer (Evans and Davies, 1999), networks in this sense are institutionalised networks (Held and McGrew, 2002). Such networks may have the functions of coordinating the work of experts and functionaries, for example within international organisations and the corporate and the NGO sector; setting policy agendas, communicating information, formulating rules, establishing and implementing policy programmes; and being mechanisms through which civil society and corporate interests are effectively embedded in the global policy process (Held and McGrew, 2002).

1.9   Structure of the book

In the following chapters, there is an overview of the different global health actors that engage in providing policy prescriptions for health care systems. The book analyses global governance in this field of health policy, and illustrates connected global policy discourses. The analysis reported is primarily based on policy documents. However, the study also includes a number of interviews with informants from the international organisations studied.

The chapters of the book illustrate a variety of global social policy actors that develop and spread ideas about health care systems. They range from international (governmental) organisations to civil society (non-governmental) actors. The positions of a number of international organisations within the UN system are highlighted, most importantly the ILO, the WHO and the World Bank (Chapter 2); and other important international organisations outside the UN system, namely the OECD and the WTO (Chapter 3). The focus then turns to the role of other important global forums where health care systems are increasingly part of the agenda, such as the G8, the G20 and the so-called BRICS (Brazil, Russia, India, China and South Africa) (Chapter 4). The hybrid organisation of the Global Fund to Fight AIDS, Tuberculosis and Malaria is considered (Chapter 5). Moving more towards the non-governmental sector, a number of civil society organisations and philanthropic organisations are discussed, most prominently the "Global Health Watch" (Chapter 6). Chapter 7 reports a case study of the application of global prescriptions to the national context, namely reforms to the Polish health care system after the end of Communism. The book concludes with a discussion about character and content of global discourses on health care systems (Chapter 8).

1.10   Contributions to the literature

The book connects to the literature on global health policy and governance in that it maps and studies global actors in health policy. By focusing on health care systems, particularly under a social policy perspective, it adds to the literature a discussion about the different meanings of health care systems and their worth beyond a focus on particular diseases or fractions of health care systems.

The book contributes to the understanding of global governance and global health governance literature (for example, Lee et al., 2002; Hein et al., 2007; Keefe and Zacher, 2008; Koivusalo and Ollila, 2008; Buse et al., 2009; Kay and Williams, 2009; Rushton and William, 2011) by discussing the application of common features of global (health) governance on the multiplicity of actors and traditional positions for the particular field of health care systems. In this context, health care systems represent not just a random example, but illuminate an ever more important issue area that is, however, little understood, because of the various meanings attached to health care systems as a topic in global health policy areas.

By including a national case study, namely Poland as a transition country, the book also links to social and health policy literature focused on national actors and institutions, and shows how transnational levels of social and health policy engage with national social policy reform processes.

2
UN Organisations: Health for All and All for Health Care Systems?

2.1 Introduction

International organisations have a key role in global discourses about various kinds of policy issues, as well as potentially influencing national social and health policymaking by other means. This is also the case with regard to concepts and prescriptions for health care systems. This chapter focuses on ideas and activities related to health care systems that have been developed by a wide array of international organisations within the UN system. It discusses respective engagements, roles, competences and power of a number of agencies within a complex and, at times, chaotic institutional setting. The chapter first introduces and discusses some of the UN bodies on more general issues of social development; namely, the UNDP, the United Nations Department of Economic and Social Affairs (UN DESA) and the Economic and Social Council (ECOSOC). The chapter then discusses the role of the WHO (section 2.4) as it tackles health care systems as part of a broader mandate to improve health globally. The shift over time in the significance of the WHO's role in questions concerning health care systems is particularly important, as it is only one expression of the difficult role the WHO is given, with great tasks and expectations, on the one hand, and notoriously limited funding, on the other. Further, the chapter considers the ILO's engagement in health care systems (section 2.7), which is particularly interesting from a historical perspective, but also in terms of most recent developments on social protection floors. The ILO's concern about health care systems is rooted in its social security mandate. The organisation may be strong in its advocacy and regulatory role; however, it is also short of resources to develop health care system concepts. The World Bank (addressed in section 2.5), in some contrast to these two "UN social agencies", has for a long time considered health policy and health care systems to be vital in encompassing approaches to fight poverty. It can draw on more significant resources, including staff working conceptually on the issues, but in this case, the differences between the different members of the World Bank Group are striking.

2.2   The United Nations' attention to health care systems: Permanent but reliable?

The "UN system" describes a group of international organisations and a package of international law. It is large and confusing in its structure. The different bodies and international organisations within this system do not all have the same status, importance, power or independence (White, 2002). Accordingly, the UN system as such does not represent a logically functioning system of global governance, even though there have been attempts to get somewhat closer to that (for example, the Report of the Secretary-General's High-Level Panel on UN System-wide Coherence (UN, 2006)). Describing the whole UN system in order to allocate the bodies and organisations concerned with health goes beyond the scope of this book. Instead, the focus is on those institutions traditionally considered in global social policy research, and identified also in other studies to play some more significant role; and on activities concerning health care systems, rather than those concerning health more generally.

The UN was established, amongst other reasons, "to cooperate in solving international economic, social, cultural and humanitarian problems and in promoting respect for human rights and fundamental freedoms; and to be a centre for harmonizing the actions of nations in attaining these ends".[1] The General Assembly is the UN's main deliberative organ, composed of the representatives of all member states, which includes most of the world's countries. Among its functions are to initiate studies and make recommendations to "promot[e] international cooperation in the economic, social, cultural, educational, and health fields" (UN Charter, Article 13; see also Articles 55, 57, 62). Any decisions, however, are taken by the representatives of the member states. UN initiatives around these health care systems issues have very limited binding character (in a legal sense); something that also applies to the UN specialised agencies working in the field (see for example White, 2002: 15ff.).

At UN General Assembly level, global health policy has predominantly taken place in the context of global development goals such as the MDGs. Three out of eight MDGs relate to health (see article 19 of the Millennium Declaration). Goal 4 relates to reducing child mortality; goal 5 to improving maternal health; and goal 6 to combating HIV/AIDS, malaria and other diseases. These MDGs were developed on the basis of the United Nations Millennium Declaration (GA A/RES/55/2), adopted in September 2000 at the United Nations Millennium Summit. Based on the fundamental principles and purposes of the UN, the MDGs go back to a set of earlier commitments made at the 1995 World Summit for Social Development in Copenhagen. Despite the lack of enforcement mechanisms for such goals, the MDGs and the connected process have gained huge importance in the foci of many global actors. It has, however, also been argued that the MDGs represent a step back in commitments already made (GASPP team, 2005; Deacon, 2007: chapter 4); and it will have to be seen if the post-2015 development agenda will mean an improvement for global health agendas, particularly concerning the issue of improving health care systems (more on this later in the chapter).

The Millennium Declaration also established a framework, and programme of work, for the entire UN system, including cooperation among the various bodies and organisations (article 30 of the Declaration). In this context, ECOSOC was supposed to be strengthened "to help it fulfil the role ascribed to it in the Charter" (article 30 of the Declaration) (for more on ECOSOC see the next section).

In 2002, the then UN secretary-general Kofi Annan commissioned the *Millennium Project*, established to develop a concrete action plan to achieve the MDGs. It concluded in 2005 with the presentation of the final recommendations and separate reports from each of the ten thematic task forces. The three task forces on the health MDGs, amongst other things, also addressed the importance of health care systems for the achievement of the respective goals. A joint statement on health care systems by the three health working groups was announced "to reflect our shared conviction that strengthening these institutions will be the key to achieving the health Millennium

Goals" (UN Millennium Project – Task Force on HIV/AIDS, 2005: xii). Despite expressed intentions and plans to do more on health care systems, there is no sign of these having been turned into action.

On the health MDGs, there have been other activities, also independent from those conducted within the Millennium Project and the UNDP, sidelining the general MDG activities. For example, in September 2007, the Global Campaign for the Health Millennium Development Goals[2] was launched, giving particular attention to the health of women and children. This consisted of several other initiatives, including the International Health Partnership (IHP) established by the UK in September 2007; the Catalytic Initiative by Canada and UNICEF in November 2007; the Results-Based Financing Initiative by Norway and the World Bank in November 2007; and the Providing for Health Initiative by Germany and France in Spring 2008. Further, the Health 8 (H8) advocating the health MDGs started in mid-2007. This was an informal group comprising the WHO, UNICEF, the United Nations Population Fund (UNFPA), the Joint UN Programme on HIV and AIDS (UNAIDS), the Global Fund, the Global Alliance for Vaccines and Immunization (GAVI), the Gates Foundation and the World Bank (see also Chapter 4). These initiatives also illustrate how different organisations network and collaborate with each other. Such activities, organisations and networks show how the two dimensions of global social policy (explained in the introduction to this book), social policy prescriptions and genuinely global social policy are not always clearly distinguishable.

At the time of writing, the MDG process is close to coming to an end. While the 2014 MDG report (UN, 2014) talks about some progress and claims that more will be done, health care systems seem to have vanished. It is only now, owing to the recent outbreak and spread of Ebola, that some are reconsidering the importance of health care systems. At the same time, new development goals, namely the SDGs, are only in the process of being developed. The outcome document of the Open Working Group for Sustainable Development Goals (OWG) proposes Goal 3 to be to "Ensure healthy lives and promote well-being for all at all ages." Under section 3.7 it says "by 2030 ensure universal access to sexual and reproductive health care services [...]" and in 3.8 "achieve universal health coverage (UHC), including financial risk protection, access to quality essential health care services, and access to safe, effective, quality, and affordable essential medicines and vaccines for all".[3] What version will eventually pass the UN General Assembly in 2015 will have to be seen.

It has to be taken into account, however, that some of the reason for the lack of (or at least varying) attention on health care systems in recent years is not only to be seen in the complexity of the issue and the limits or character of globally applicable development goals. It was also the economic and financial crisis of 2008 and following global and regional crises of different kinds that made the world community focus on other fields and policies. Development aid, including to the health sector, broke down in the past few years as a consequence of the crisis, despite frequent calls that this should not happen. For example, at a high-level consultation in Geneva in January 2009, there was a strong call for solidarity between governments and citizens in the sense of "sharing risks and responsibilities as a basis of strong health care systems" (section 8). The outcome document of that event further summarised: "the financial crisis has provoked an examination of the values that underpin societies worldwide. The health response should likewise aim to be transformative and promote a focus on social justice" (section 10).[4] Most recent OECD data shows an increase in aid levels.[5] However, it will have to be seen if that marks a turn, particularly given that the crisis is not considered to be fully overcome, and significant inequalities continue to characterise the relationships between people within and across countries.

2.3   UN Economic and Social Council (ECOSOC), UNDP, UN DESA

The UN, apart from being a system of international organisations (some of which I will turn to later in this chapter), also has some functional bodies. One of them is ECOSOC, responsible for developing the UN's economic and social policies. ECOSOC serves as a forum for the discussion of international economic and social issues and formulates policy recommendations to member states and the UN system. Its mission includes the attainment of "identifying solutions to international economic, social and health problems".[6] It has also been designated as the principal organ to coordinate the economic, social and related work between the UN specialised agencies and commissions, including, originally, the MDGs. In fact, despite having been created as one of the six main bodies of the UN, it was placed under the authority of the UN General Assembly (UN Charter Article 60), which means it has not been given any decision-making power. Further, the other UN agencies are not forced to abide by the ECOSOC's recommendations and decisions. This has generated a permanent debate regarding the desirable role of the ECOSOC in global health governance (for example, Martens, 2005; South Centre, 2006).

Regarding health, ECOSOC's activities have included a High-Level Segment on the Contribution of Human Resources Development in 2002 that, amongst other things, paid attention to the fields of health and education more broadly. Preparing this, three one-day round-table discussions took place prior to the High-Level Segment, one of them entitled Health and Development (chaired by Gro Harlem Brundtland).[7] The round table itself addressed health care systems as an important issue to development. However, health care systems did not prominently feature in the Ministerial Declaration following this event. The only vague points of reference were a reaffirmation of "the need to provide access to effective and equitable primary health-care systems in all communities" (section 10). Instead, health was put into another context, stating that "[e]fforts should continue to ensure improved access to medicines and affordable health systems in line with the Agreement on Trade-Related Intellectual Property Rights and public health adopted at the fourth WTO ministerial conference held at Doha" (article 11; see also Chapter 3). Also in other similar meetings, facilitated by ECOSOC, such as the high-level segment for representatives from member states, official pronouncements after the meetings often include a short statement about the importance of health care systems when discussions concern development policy, reaching the MDGs and so on. However, there is no explicit or extensive further engagement from the side of the organisation with the issue.

United Nations Development Programme (UNDP)

UNDP serves as the UN's global development network. Its purpose is to "advocat[e] for change and connect [...] countries to knowledge, experience and resources to help people build a better life".[8] Similarly to ECOSOC, the UNDP does not have a health mandate as such. However, as it has been made responsible for the process of reaching the MDGs, and is now supposed to continue that role with the SDGs, health is among the issues of concern. This has involved work on health issues as connected to the particular health MDGs; however, health care systems as an important context for these issues seem to have been neglected.

Some health-connected activity has come from the UNDP staff concerning global public goods (Kaul et al., 1999, 2003). Nevertheless, health care systems have not been of major concern here either. In setting up agendas and to some extent coordinating UN-wide activities, organisations such as ECOSOC and UNDP would have some power to shift attention to health care system issues; given their limited size and resources, and a very broad agenda of topics to deal with, these organisations have not, though, significantly contributed to making health care systems a key issue.

United Nations Department for Economic and Social Affairs (UN DESA)

Another such body is UN DESA.[9] It is responsible for supporting international cooperation on development and national agenda-setting and decision-making on development issues. UN DESA's work is primarily geared to implementing the Copenhagen Declaration, with particular attention to poverty eradication, employment generation and social integration. This translates into analytical and statistical work on related issues, as well as in assistance to developing countries and transition countries in organising their socio-economic development. Particularly, UN DESA's Division of Social Policy and Development is concerned with social policy issues. Health care systems do not get the attention they would deserve, as with UNDP and ECOSOC. For example, while the first Report on the World Social Situation (UN DESA, 1957) contained a full chapter on health, this was significantly shorter in the one to follow, and for the recent reports there are only selected sentences on health care systems.[10] Nevertheless, Social Policy Guidance Notes (Ortiz, 2007) have been prepared, and these include a section on health care systems.

Conclusions

ECOSOC, UNDP and UN DESA occasionally touch upon health care systems, usually in the context of development policy or, more specifically, in the process of working towards fulfilling the MDGs, but they have not given it a prominent place in their activities and coordinative functions within the UN. Most pronouncements appear, instead, in the form of short political statements. While that is, perhaps, not surprising regarding the function and size of these bodies, and the breadth of global topics they are covering, it is still worrying given the repeated statements and common knowledge about the centrality of health systems in the contexts of development and human well-being.

The case is different for some of the specialised UN "social" agencies and IFIs, which are international organisations in their own right with separate councils, assemblies, secretariats, budgets and so on that deal with global and national health matters, such as WHO, the World Bank and ILO, which are discussed in the following sections.

2.4 WHO as the world's health care system organisation?

Within the UN system or family of international organisations, there is one organisation that is explicitly devoted to health – the WHO. The constitution of the WHO provides the organisation with a norm-setting and a coordinative mandate. The most basic objective is to work for the "attainment by all people of the highest possible level of health", which includes, among the WHO's functions, to assist governments in strengthening their health services (Constitution of the WHO, article 2c). Obviously, attempting to fulfil that has been a challenge throughout the WHO's history. Amongst other things, this can be seen through the changing self-description: from a "world conscience" (WHA, 1973) to a "health advocate" (WHO, 1998) to a "directing and coordinating authority in international health work" (WHO, 2006: 1). In the World Health Report 2010, the WHO states:

> Health financing is an important part of broader efforts to ensure social protection in health. As such, WHO is joint lead agency with the ILO in the United Nations initiative to help countries develop a comprehensive Social Protection Floor, which includes the type of financial risk protection [...] and the broader aspects of income replacement and social support in the event of illness.[11]

The latest account of the WHO's role and functions has been provided in the form of its twelfth general programme of work, adopted by the World Health Assembly in May 2013. Here, the WHO presents itself much more pragmatically, referring to its "unique legitimacy as an evidence-based multilateral agency to articulate six leadership priorities that provide programmatic direction and two additional priorities that reflect the governance and managerial dimensions of reform" (WHO, 2014).

On health care systems in particular, the WHO's constitution contains the basic idea that "[g]overnments have a responsibility for the health of their peoples which can be fulfilled only by the provision of adequate health and social measures" (Constitution of the WHO). The WHO has made significant efforts to turn this health system-related mandate into a meaningful role. The organisation has, for a long time, provided knowledge about, and advice on, health care systems. In a historical perspective, we can observe cyclical changes with regard to the relative importance given to the topic of health care systems at different times. Furthermore, the WHO has continuously struggled to find the right expressions for its role, and has tried to develop strategies, mechanisms and information channels to fulfil a health-system mandate.

Certainly, the WHO secretariat has used international gatherings in the form of conferences or the annual World Health Assemblies of the WHO's member states for the purpose of disseminating particular conceptual and normative models, and of facilitating policy learning (potentially leading to policy transfer). Other important instrumental tools are publications, most prominently the annual World Health Reports; and health data collected, prepared and disseminated by the WHO. An additional instrument that the WHO used is specialised commissions of international experts that focus on particular issues of interest.

A number of different terms and concepts used to refer to health care systems can be found when looking for related work and activity at WHO. These conceptual tools include the "Primary Health Care" (PHC) approach and the "Health for All" (HFA) strategy; the World Health Report 2000s understanding of health care systems (functions); health system financing; social health insurance; health system strengthening; the diagonal approach and Universal Health Coverage (UHC). The main emphasis regarding which concept to use has changed over time, while all of them have been more or less carried through the related debates and publications ever since they were "invented". These conceptual shifts are also observable in the broader global health debates (including among other global actors). Approaching such changes in historical sequences (though naturally some thoughts and initiatives have also been developed in parallel), the following sections trace the development and the up and downs of the WHO's health care system-related activities, starting from the 1970s.

The PHC approach and the HFA strategy were developed in the context of the Alma-Ata Conference and the Alma-Ata Declaration (WHO/UNICEF, 1978) in the 1970s. The Alma-Ata Declaration starts from the notion that health inequalities are considered to be a problem in all countries and develops its ideas accordingly. It is normatively based on the idea of health as a fundamental human right, and "the attainment of the highest possible level of health [...] [as] a most important world-wide social goal whose realization requires the action of many other social and economic sectors in addition to the health sector" (WHO/UNICEF, 1978: I). Connected to this is the HFA principle. On defining health care systems, the Alma-Ata Declaration marked the first attempt to introduce basic principles for health care systems, accompanied by a model of the organisation of health care systems. It introduced the PHC approach that is "in the spirit of social justice" (WHO/UNICEF, 1978: V). This PHC model envisaged an important role and responsibility regarding the health of the people to be realised by the state or govern-ment through the provision of adequate health and social measures (WHO/UNICEF, 1978: V). Governments were, accordingly, recom-mended to develop national policies, strategies and plans of action for primary health care within a comprehensive national health care system (WHO/UNICEF, 1978: VIII). Following Kickbusch (2000: 981), this did not only give governments the responsibility for the health of their people, but "was no less than a redefinition of the norms and expectations of the state role in regard to health". However, the Alma-Ata Declaration does not only focus on the role of the state, but also states that "people have the right and duty to participate individually and collectively in the planning and implementation of their health care" (WHO/UNICEF, 1978: IV). The Alma-Ata Declaration does not define health care systems, but primary health care as

essential health care based on practical, scientifically sound and socially acceptable methods and technology made universally accessible to individuals and families in the community through their full participation and at a cost that the community and country can afford to maintain at every stage of their development in the spirit of self-reliance and self-determination. It forms an integral part both of the country's health system, of which it is the central function and main focus, and of the overall social and economic development of the community. It is the first level of contact of individuals, the family and community with the national health system bringing health care as close as possible to where people live and work, and constitutes the first element of a continuing health care process.

(WHO/UNICEF, 1978: VI)

What many international health experts, from within the WHO as well as representatives from CSOs, enthusiastically celebrated and believed to represent an important new role for the organisation in supporting health care systems in a socially acceptable way, soon provoked, at least partly, the formulation of alternative models. At the level of ideas, differences have been identified regarding the support of so-called comprehensive Primary Health Care approaches, usually connected to the WHO and other UN social agencies, and those of selective health approaches, associated with UNICEF and the IFIs (see for example Koivusalo and Ollila, 1997). Vertical approaches are, in their "pure" form, programmes or interventions that concentrate on a single disease and are usually organised independently. In contrast, horizontal approaches encompass several health interventions within a more comprehensive primary care approach (see for example Victora et al., 2004). Walsh and Warren (1980), for instance, have argued for selective PHC because they say it "cannot be overemphasized that the greatest immediate efforts in health care in less developed areas should be aimed at preventing and managing those few diseases that cause the greatest mortality and morbidity and for which there are medical interventions of relatively high efficacy" (Walsh and Warren, 1980: 146). They do this with regard to the Alma-Ata Declaration that had clearly called for a comprehensive, horizontal approach in health. However, health care systems per se cannot be fully equated with horizontal approaches – rather, periods of interest in horizontal approaches have provided a platform for engaging with health care systems more thoroughly (see also the Commission on the Social Determinants of Health, following). In recent years, the focus has shifted to the concept of Universal Health Coverage. One expression of this was the foundation of a Joint Learning Network in 2010.[12] Among the funders were the WHO, the Gates Foundation, the ILO and the World Bank. Discussions about the topic also emerged in World Bank blogs; for example, Adam Wagstaff argued:

> The problem with [...] much if not most of the debate on universal coverage is that it portrays the universal health coverage challenge as an either-or problem. People either have coverage or they don't. In actual fact, everyone everywhere has some coverage. The stark reality, though, is that in many – if not most – countries there are larger inequalities in coverage, typically mirroring pretty closely the income distribution. [...] The challenge, it seems to me, is [...] really about narrowing inequalities in coverage.[13]

The Rockefeller Foundation concluded in a report that "the cost of transitioning towards universal health coverage may be lower than assumed. This applies both in the expansion phase and the subsequent deepening of coverage" (Rockefeller Foundation, 2010: 7). The topic became the subject of an International Forum on Universal Health Coverage (Mexico, 1–2 April 2012); but more important was that the 65th session of the World Health Assembly in May 2012 included universal health coverage as a key issue.[14] Following events, such as the Global Symposium on Health System Research (Beijing, 2012) and subsequent World Health Assemblies gave ever more attention to the issue.[15] Related reports explained

> [m]oving towards universal coverage is a process that needs progress on several fronts: the range of services that are available to people (consisting of medicines, medical products, health workers, infrastructure and information required to ensure good quality); the proportion of the costs of those services that are covered; and the proportion of the population that is covered. These gains need to be protected during financial or economic downturns. Universal health coverage is not about achieving a fixed minimum package.
>
> (WHO EB, 2013)

Last but not least, the World Health Report 2013 was dedicated to "Research for Universal Health Coverage" (WHO, 2013).[16]

Parallel to these advances, the WHO generated basic models and developed indicators upon which it collects data that monitors and reports the state of the world's health care systems. In the second half of the 1990s, for example, the WHO undertook major activities in relation to advising national health care systems, culminating in the World Health Report 2000 on health systems (WHO, 2000). For this specific topic, the ball was set rolling by the countries of the Non-Aligned Movement (NAM), which presented a proposal on strengthening health care system development in developing countries; this was adopted by the World Health Assembly (WHA) (resolution WHA50.27), resulting in a plan of action (as called for in resolution EB100.RB1). Following this, an ad hoc group for health care system development was put into place, as well as an external advisory group to examine the plan of action for the global initiative. While the World Health Report 1999 Making a Difference (WHO, 1999) concerned the WHO's role, the World Health Report 2000 conceptualised, defined and elaborated the importance and meaning of health care systems.

More concretely, the World Health Report 2000 commences with the assumption that every country has a health care system, though their respective performance may be different. It mentions fragmentation of health care systems, describing that countries usually have "no single health care system, but several distinct health financing and provision subsystems, embracing different types of traditional and alternative practice, as well as public, private and not-for-profit hospitals and clinics, sometimes offering services for limited population subgroups" (WHO, 1999: 31). The World Health Report 1999, on the other hand, is more pragmatic, summarising health care systems as aiming to achieve the following: improving health status; reducing health inequalities; enhancing responsiveness to legitimate expectations; increasing efficiency; protecting individuals, families and communities from financial loss; and enhancing fairness in the financing and delivery of care (WHO, 1999: 32–33). According to the World Health Report 2000, health care systems should guarantee the "best attainable coverage level – goodness" and at the same time the "smallest feasible differences among individuals and groups – fairness" (WHO, 2000: 26).

In terms of definitions, the World Health Report 2000 describes health care systems as "comprising all the organizations, institutions and resources that are devoted to producing health actions", while health actions are "any effort, whether in personal health care, public health services or through inter-sectoral initiatives whose primary purpose is to improve health" (WHO, 2000: xi). In order to operationalize health care systems and develop measurable indicators accordingly, the World Health Report 2000 distinguishes four functions of health care systems: service provision, resource generation, financing and stewardship.[17]

The WHO's approach in general is intended to apply to all countries (Murray and Evans, 2003a: 5). That may take different shapes, though, and concrete recommendations or different forms of policy models to particular groups of countries. Regarding the Alma-Ata ideas, it is interesting to see how much of the discussion is connected to developing countries, while in practice it has perhaps been most effective in the European region. Also, the World Health Report 2000, in some cases, distinguishes between countries when it does not appear easily possible to realise concepts such as big risk pools in particular settings.

Health care provision is considered the core function of health care systems. The World Health Report 2000 supports a public-private mix, but there is no clear statement about the desirable degree of (de)centralisation. Concerning the financing of health care systems, the report states that it is not the question of public versus private sources of financing that matters, but that of pre-payment versus out-of-pocket payments (including user fees). Different forms of insurance systems are considered more realistic than a universal tax-based system. Pools should add up to comprehensive redistributive systems, and financing should be organised in a centralised way. The role of the state in regulation, finally, should be – according to the stewardship model – that of defining the vision and direction of health care systems, regulating the relationships between the different elements of health care systems, and generating and providing information on health care system-related issues. Accordingly, the World Health Report 2000 proposes a system of universal access with a prepayment system (taxation or insurance), fairly distributed pre-payments and strategic purchasing. The content of the benefit package should be decided upon by an explicit, public process of priority setting.

At the time when the World Health Report 2000 was published, the WHO was quite euphoric about its "new role", which was supposed to be marked and initiated by its report. Through this new focus, the WHO had attempted to "restore its position as an international expert leader in the field of health" (Taipale, 2000: 1). Nevertheless, the reaction to the report by some member states and academics has not helped or furthered the position of the WHO and its work on health care systems. The literature on the topic includes severe criticism about the indicators used to assess health care systems and the resulting rankings (for example, Ollila and Koivusalo, 2000, 2002; Navarro, 2001). Thus, instead of a strengthened WHO with a new role as global health leader, other organisations (such as the World Bank and the OECD) gained strength as a consequence of the WHO's failings. While within the WHO that criticism was acknowledged and considered to some extent (see Murray and Evans, 2003b), subsequently it had to withdraw from further rankings and major analytical activity in the field, owing to the withdrawal of support by some of its member states. At the same time, other member states have continued to request health care system analyses by the WHO as repeatedly mentioned in WHO reports (for example, Murray and Evans, 2003b; WHO, 2007a). A couple of years later, the issue of monitoring has come up again – but perhaps rather more humbly compared with what had been attempted with the World Health Report 2000:

> A monitoring system for health systems strengthening needs to capture trends in health system inputs and outputs, supported by coverage data with a small set of indicators. Progress can be summarized with a country "dashboard" that includes key indicators for these core areas and describes progress on an annual or bi-annual basis. The dashboard should also provide contextual information such as the country health situation in relation to its level of economic development or health expenditure.
>
> (WHO CHM, 2007a: 20)

The Commission on Macroeconomics and Health (CMH) is also noteworthy in this context. The CMH worked from 2000 to 2001, and brought together some of the world's top economists, headed by Jeffrey Sachs.[18] It released its final report in 2001 (WHO CMH, 2001). The CMH's final report (WHO CMH, 2001) is thematically situated within the context of poverty and the world's poor people, related economic growth and long-term economic development within countries. The investments in health are said to "work best as part of a sound overall development strategy", including an "active role of government in [...] ensuring core investments in health, [...] guaranteeing the rule of law..." (WHO CMH, 2001: 25–26). Health care systems in developing countries are described as being strained and requiring more resources (including potential donor resources) (WHO CMH, 2001: 39), but there is no further definition of health care systems as such. According to this focus on the poor, the CMH report discusses the minimum of health provision, as a starting point for the countries and people in focus (WHO CMH, 2001: 56), and thus its estimates and recommendations are based on this idea of a rather minimal health care system for the purpose of poverty reduction (WHO CMH, 2001: 56). The CMH does not provide for prescriptions regarding a more advanced health care system model. In that sense, the CMH proposes community financing schemes that are financed from contributions, tax revenues and foreign assistance. There should be universal coverage, at least, to this very narrow benefit package, defined by national government and covering the major communicable diseases and maternal and childcare. The relevance and implications of this commission have been differently regarded and assessed. Seidel (2003: 117) states that "[a]lthough encompassing not entirely the volume and the originality of work that characterised the preparation of the World Bank's annual World Development Report 1993 Investing in Health, the report of the Commission on Macroeconomics and Health constitutes a landmark and reference point for the international health policy discussion and the relative importance of health within development assistance". There is also evidence that the CMH's descriptions and recommendations had important implications for how economists look at health care systems (see for example Hsiao and Heller, 2007). Others however, such as Banerji (2002: 733), have severely criticised the CMH's composition and work as "ahistorical, apolitical and atheoretical".

Commission on Social Determinants of Health (CSDH)

From 2005 to 2008, the CSDH worked on the social determinants of health.[19] It had been appointed by the then director-general Lee Jong-Wook and comprised a number of working groups with members from academia, practitioners, civil society representatives and so on. The work also importantly included health care systems (as social determinants of health). The CSDH approached health care systems within a broad concept of the social determinants of health and the context of tackling health inequities. Health care systems are regarded and treated as one determinant of health. This includes a focus on rights and universal access to health care (and related commodities, such as clean water and sanitation). The CSDH's recommendations take up the Alma-Ata declaration's PHC model. The emphasis is on the public sector, particularly public financing (ideally a taxation system), while for provision the CSDH acknowledged that there are also acceptable private providers in place. However, it does not go into detail with the specific mix. The dimensions of financing and provision are not always clearly differentiated. The state is given an important role and ultimate responsibility in the regulation of health care systems, but other levels, actors and civil society are also considered as crucial in decision-making. The proposed strategies for Ministries of Health (WHO CSDH, 2007: 24) show a process focus, which opens the space for context-specific health care system arrangements. When the Health Systems Knowledge Network of the WHO CSDH released its final report, "Challenging Inequity Through Health Systems", in June 2007, health systems were said to be understood as "all activities whose primary purpose is to improve health" (WHO Commission on the Social Determinants of Health, 2007: v), and the report focused on a discussion of how health care systems can address health inequity. The focus, however, was not only on providing knowledge, but also creating a "social movement for health equity" (Marmot et al., 2012: 181).

In 2006, the WHO's secretariat made a new effort to elaborate a strategy for strengthening health care systems, which was accompanied by a new cluster of "Health Systems and Services". Following, the WHO (2007: 27) attempted to develop the idea of a "diagonal" approach with the following characteristics: taking the desired health outcomes as the starting point for identifying health care system constraints; meeting specific health outcomes simultaneously with supporting system-wide effects and other programmes; primarily addressing health care system policy and capacity issues; encouraging comprehensive national health sector strategies and plans; and monitoring and evaluating health care systems.

One attempt to get further in health care system issues was made in 2008, when WHO and the World Bank organised a session to discuss the issue of health care systems and vertical health initiatives. Echoing the idea of "diagonal" approaches and the related report on the expert consultation regarding positive synergies between health care systems and Global Health Initiatives (WHO, 2008b), Carissa Etienne,[20] the then WHO assistant director-general for/of Health Systems and Services, said: "It is not about choosing between health system strengthening on the one hand and disease-specific programmes on the other. It is about working together to generate added value."[21]

Around the same time, one could observe a move back to PHC in the form of the World Health Report 2008 Primary Health Care – Now More Than Ever (WHO, 2008c).[22] The World Health Report 2008 states that

> Moving towards health for all requires that health systems respond to the challenges of a changing world and growing expectations for better performance. This involves substantial reorientation and reform of the ways health systems operate in society today: those reforms constitute the agenda for the renewal of PHC.
>
> (WHO, 2008c: xii)

The report continues to emphasise the "recognition that providing a sense of direction to health systems requires a set of specific and context-sensitive reforms that respond to the health challenges of today and prepare for those of tomorrow" (WHO, 2008c: xiv). What is then offered are four groups of PHC reforms, namely universal coverage reforms, service delivery reforms, public policy reforms and leadership reforms.

Meanwhile, health care system *strengthening* came into focus. The WHO released "Systems thinking for health systems strengthening", which argues that "we must know the system in order to strengthen it – and from that base we can design better interventions and evaluations, for both health care systems strengthening interventions and for interventions targeting specific diseases or conditions but with the potential of having system-wide effects" (Alliance for Health Policy and Systems Research and WHO, 2009). In order to achieve this, the report proposes "Ten Steps to Systems Thinking for real-world guidance in applying such an approach to the health system." Instead of discussing different health care system models, these ten steps are more "organisational", in the sense of reflecting on how to engage stakeholders, how to approach collective brainstorming, how to develop plans and so on.

It is important to note that we can observe a number of parallel debates, all addressing health care systems and their functions, amongst other things under the topic of "social health insurance" (WHO, 2009b), or relating to "health system financing" (WHO, 2010; see also Lee and Goodman, 2002). Despite all these attempts made to function as a "health-system organisation", WHO's performance is clearly not straightforwardly convincing. We are faced with a multiple, ambitious, but also ambiguous mandate that the WHO has over several decades struggled to translate into a convincing role in guiding national health care systems. The aftermath of the global economic and financial crisis that started in 2007/2008, the latest from 2012, let the WHO's voice in this field become stunted. That only added to the criticisms following the publication of the World Health Report 2000. Therefore, concluding this rough historical sketch of the WHO's engagement with health care systems, it can be seen that no one coherent model or set of prescriptions has developed out of a specific mandate given to the organisation. Nevertheless, a couple of general features from WHO health care system prescriptions can be drawn: WHO approaches are usually characterised by a universal approach in the sense that they are supposed to apply to and inform all countries (with the exception of the CMH which was explicitly for low-income countries). All documents generally reject user fees; however, some categorically reject them, while others consider them not to be desirable (except in cases of over-utilisation). For example, the World Health Report 2000 implies that it might not be easy just to abolish user fees without a sound means of substituting the missing revenue.

Nevertheless, the differences between the ideational stream of an Alma-Ata Declaration and that of the World Health Report 2000 are important. While the former develops a model out of concern about inequities in health, the latter pursues a rather more technical goal of defining, in detail, the functions, elements and options of health care systems in a generalised way. The Alma-Ata Declaration introduces the so-called PHC model, giving the state a central role in the development of national health policies with regard to PHC and the broader health care system. While the World Health Report

2000 approached health care systems in an all-encompassing sense and distinguished functions (provision, resource generation, financing and stewardship), the PHC model is more focused on levels of care (provision) and decision-making processes.

2.5 World Bank

Introduction

The WHO has hardly been alone in its concern about and attempt to provide health care system prescriptions. For a number of reasons, mainly caused by the combination of the weakness of the WHO's work and the nature of health as a complex policy field, there is multi-actor action on various health matters. Health care systems are not an exception here, and the World Bank has for a long time been the other key global health actor. From its general mission to fight poverty and improve living standards in the developing world (see Articles of Agreement of the International Bank for Reconstruction and Development (IBRD) and the International Development Association (IDA)), the World Bank has argued it had a mandate in health care system matters. In practice, it is strategy papers by which the World Bank justifies and defines such an engagement. The World Bank's activities encompass a range of things, including lending and project activities, but also important research and policy advice.

Health was not an initial, or primary, mandate of the World Bank, and concern about the sector has evolved out of the insight that it was an important factor when supporting a country's development, in the context of poverty alleviation. The World Bank's engagement has increased since the 1980s, not only in scale, but also in how comprehensively health care systems have been understood. The first major contribution in terms of ideas was the World Development Report 1993, which provoked a number of controversial debates, for example on user fees and privatisation (see for example Brugha and Zwi, 2002). The World Bank's take on the issue, focus and ideas have changed and concretised since then. Besides issues of inequity and lacking access to health services for some groups of the population, World Bank work (for example, World Bank, 1993) has also been concerned with the misallocation of public money, inefficiency and expanding health costs.

Looking at the organisation's mandate, the engagement of the World Bank in health issues is connected to, and in the context of, its commitment to fighting poverty. Accordingly, its policy models and advice are usually tailored or applied to low- and middle-income countries, and with an implicit or explicit focus on poor people. The goals or principles of the World Bank's health care system activities are, thus, deeply grounded in the alleviation of poverty and the provision of services to poor people. More encompassing reflections and models of health care systems can be found in some less prominent publications through the World Bank and may serve as background material.

At the same time, it is obvious that, owing to the rising number of global actors in various health fields and limited resources, the World Bank – like the WHO – has seen an increased need to justify its role in the field and its focus of activity within it. While the Bank in 1997 was satisfied with explaining its comparative advantage by its "global experience and ability to combine country-specific research and analysis with the mobilization of significant financial resources across many sectors" (World Bank, 1997), the 2007 strategy is much more detailed about this issue and lists: an intersectoral and systems approach to country assistance, which allows the Bank to engage at national and subnational level with all government sectors but particularly ministries of finance; its capacity for large-scale implementation of projects and programmes including its financial management and procurement system for large-scale operations; its multiple financing instrumental and products; its global nature allowing facilitation of interregional sharing of experience; its core economic and fiscal analysis capacity across all sectors; its substantial country focus and presence; engaging private health actors through both the Bank (IBRD and IDA) and the IFC; health care system development and strengthening (but not in every aspect of it). In particular, regarding health care system performance, the comparative advantages are summarised as follows: health financing (for example, level and source of funding, health insurance organisation and regulation, health service contracting and provider payment mechanisms); system governance; accountability for health service delivery; and demand side intervention (for example, conditional cash transfers to boost demand for health interventions, communities' and consumers' voice and choice in the delivery of health services) (World Bank, 2007: 17–18).

The following sections address the understanding of health care systems as expressed in World Bank documents, with a particular attention to the functions of provision, financing and regulation.

The World Bank's concept of health care systems

To some extent in contrast to the WHO's World Health Report 2000, the World Bank's publications are less concerned about what a health care system *is* (in terms of definition) than what it should achieve. This is best exemplified by the following quote from its revised Health, Nutrition and Population (HNP) strategy paper that does, in its main part, not even try to define health care systems but focuses on strengthening health systems:

> "Strengthening health systems" may sound abstract and less important than specific disease control technology [...] But, well-organized and sustainable health systems are necessary to achieve results. [...] Strengthening health systems is not a result in itself. Success cannot be claimed until the right chain of events on the ground prevents avoidable deaths and extreme financial hardship due to illness because, without results, health system strengthening has no meaning. However, without health system strengthening, there will be no results.
>
> (World Bank, 2007: 14)

Looking at the past decade or so, the World Bank documents describe the context of health care systems (with the focus on low- and middle-income countries), or the problems that require health action, usually making one or several of the following points: the private sector is dominant in most low-income countries and many middle-income countries; this includes private service delivery; however, there is also private funding via household out-of-pocket spending; multiple and fragmented forums of risk pooling arrangements coexist; and low participation in risk pooling in low income countries and among the poor (in middle-income countries in the informal sector and among the self-employed) (for example, World Bank, 2007: section 51, 81, Annex L). When addressing health care systems, their strengthening is, for the focus of the Bank's work, not a policy objective in itself, and needs to be linked with a country's fiscal policy and competitiveness (World Bank, 2007: section 36).

The significance of strengthened health care systems is only expressed in the context of improving health and the financial protection in relation to the costs of illness (World Bank, 2007: 14). section 106 of the paper summarises:

> A well-organized and sustainable health system is essential to achieve financial protection by preventing the impoverishing effects of health shocks (for example, through health insurance) and mitigating their effects. An efficient public financing and pro-poor subsidy policy in the health sector, access to effective financial risk-pooling mechanisms (for example, health insurance), and household access to borrowing through better financial market environments are among the interventions that can help improve financial protection. Client countries face options in organizing risk pooling, including general tax-based systems, social insurance systems (financed out of payroll-tax contributions), and/or private health insurance arrangements, including not-for-profit community health insurance.

Referring to the WHO's World Health Report 2000, the strategy paper *defines* health care systems as "encompass[ing] all country activities, organisations, governance arrangements and resources (public and private) dedicated to improving and maintaining, or restoring the health of individuals and populations and/ or prevent households from falling into poverty (or becoming further impoverished) as a result of illness" (World Bank, 2007: section 15; see also section 84). They are further described as "adaptive systems", comprising four main functions: stewardship (regulation), health service provision, health financing and health service input (World Bank, 2007: 169 (Annex L)).

In general, the 2007 strategy gives governments the responsibility to "ensure people's access to essential services and financial protection [by] rais[ing] stable, sufficient, long-term public and private financial resources, predictable, equitable, efficient and in a way that minimizes economic distortions" (World Bank, 2007: section 112). While not describing *provision* as the most important function (in contrast to the World Health Report 2000), the health strategy paper calls "[p]ublic and private health service provision [...] the most *visible* product of the health care system" (World Bank, 2007: 169; emphasis added). As in the earlier strategy paper (World Bank, 1997), a public-private mix in provision is understood to be the reality in individual countries and has to be developed into a coherent system. The World Development Report 2004 states that "[t]here is no presumption that one type of provider – public, for-profit, or not-for-profit – is likely to be better than any other" (World Bank, 2003: 151), and the 2007 HNP sector strategy paper describes the World Bank's role in providing policy models for health care provision as follows:

> Bank advisory capacity on health system strengthening needs to be able to provide sound, feasible, and sustainable advice on when and how to invest in in-house public service delivery infrastructure or contract out with the private sector (for-profit and not-for-profit) in LICs and MICs.
>
> (World Bank, 2007: section 82)

Referring to the common call to decentralisation in service provision, the World Development Report 2004 points to the mixed results of decentralised health service provision:

> Transferring the provision function to local governments has often overwhelmed them, leaving them with little capacity and incentives to develop the policy function and encourage citizen oversight.
>
> (World Bank, 2003: 147)

Regarding the financing function, some publications (for example, Gwatkin et al., 2005; Yazbeck, 2006) argue that health services primarily benefit the better off, and thus propose that public spending should only be on the poor. However, the 2007 strategy paper appears to be indifferent concerning the question of public or private financing:

> Household out-of-pocket private funding dominates health financing in LICs and in many MICs. [...] Thus, improving financial protection requires the Bank to provide sound policy advice to

client countries not only about the best use of DAH[23] but also how to pool household out-of-pocket expenditures for the non-poor so that household demand and insurers (public and/or private) offer better pooling of financial risk. In the same context, user fees have a role to play as copayment when there is evidence of excess demand.

(World Bank, 2007: section 104, footnote added)

The paper continues by affirming that there is no support for one specific approach, no "one-size-fits-all blueprint for organizing risk pooling across countries" (World Bank, 2007: section 109). There is also a differentiation for proposed action with regard to low-income countries (LICs) and middle-income countries (MICs). While for LICs the three challenges are said to be expanding participation in risk pooling, solving the development assistance for health (DAH) volatility problem, and ensuring sufficient economic growth, the challenges to MICs read differently: "fiscal sustainability linked to systemic efficiency and potential challenges from past decisions linking social health insurance financing to labor status. The insurance-labor link can distort labor markets and labor costs through the use of payroll taxes as the main revenue-raising mechanism for social health insurance" (World Bank, 2007: section 113). In this strategy paper, we also find a more critical stance concerning the question of the usefulness of decentralisation in health financing than in previous publications.

Provision

Initially, the Bank became engaged in the field of health through its work on population policies. A formal health policy was adopted in 1974, and more concrete ideas were formulated in the World Development Report 1980 (World Bank, 1980b), linking problems of health and malnutrition to poverty, and arguing for a greater emphasis on social sector lending (Ruger, 2005). At the same time, the 1980 Health Sector Policy Paper (World Bank, 1980a) provided a first rationale for investments in the health sector. This paper introduced a system of basic health services with three levels: community health workers, a second level facility (a rural health centre, an urban clinic or a small district hospital) and a third level in the shape of a referral hospital. While the report was detailed regarding the provision function, it was much less so on financing: "the proposals for financing health care services go into little detail, are on the optimistic side (the resources on health were forecast to increase over the following two decades [...] vague, and even unrealistic (for example local insurance systems, or for cooperatives responsible for importing and distributing essential drugs)" (Brunet-Jailly, 1999: 349).

While an actor-mix in health care provision is the option, the stress used to be more on the advantages of private providers and decentralisation (via District Hospitals) (World Bank, 1993). The 1997 Strategy Paper (World Bank, 1997) continued with the idea of a mix; however, concrete models are not discussed. The 2007 strategy paper (World Bank, 2007) also promotes the mix, but here it is particularly concerned with the importance of building up a coherent system. The World Development Report 2004 had made explicit that neither type of provider (public or private) would be regarded as better as such, and had expressed caution about decentralisation in service provision.

Financing

In the second half of the 1980s, a shift towards interest in the financing function of health care systems occurred. A study entitled Financing Health Services in Developing Countries: An Agenda for Reform (World Bank, 1987) went further into the topic (see for example Brunet-Jailly, 1999; Ruger, 2005). At that time, the perception was that "public spending in general cannot be increased; indeed, in many countries, it must be curtailed" (World Bank, 1987: 1, quoted in Brunet-Jailly, 1999). Accordingly, the idea was that public money could be saved by only paying for health services for the poor (see Brunet-Jailly, 1999: 350).

A widely taken-up and critically discussed publication of the World Bank has been the World Development Report 1993: Investing in Health (World Bank, 1993). The health-system related problems of poor countries are described here as the misallocation of public money, inequity and lack of access for the poor, inefficiency (wasted money) and exploding health costs (World Bank, 1993: 3). The report proposes a strong reliance on private providers (for example, faith-based NGOs or private doctors) that are said to be often more efficient than public providers. Government involvement would be necessary where it increased the supply of public goods. The District Hospital is suggested as the best organisational level for service provision.

Regarding health-system financing, the World Development Report 1993 proposes to reduce government expenditure on tertiary health care facilities and specialist provision. Instead, governments should finance, implement and ensure the delivery of a package of public health interventions. Public subsidies "if they mainly benefit the wealthy, should be phased out during a transitional period" (World Bank, 1993: 7). The remaining services should be financed privately, or through public or private health insurance to be promoted and regulated by governments. More concretely, the report calls for less public spending on less cost-effective interventions, and instead suggested the doubling or tripling of spending on basic public health programmes. The report further promotes some degree of targeting (instead of universal provision) and user fees, as applicable. Administrative and budgetary responsibility should further be organised in a decentralised way. Summarising with regard to the provision and financing of health care, this means the "[p]rovision of cost-effective health services to the poor is an effective and socially acceptable approach to poverty reduction. Most countries view access to basic health care as a basic human right" (World Bank, 1993: 5). On the regulatory responsibilities of the state, the report describes highly centralised decision-making as problematic (regarding the hospital sector) (World Bank, 1993: 4). Nevertheless, "[g]overnments have an important role to play in regulating privately provided health insurance, in order to ensure widespread coverage and hold down costs" (World Bank, 1993: 5). Governments are responsible for defining the benefit package according to cost-effectiveness measurements, namely disability-adjusted life years (DALYs). Further criteria are: mother and child care, family planning services, tuberculosis control, STDs control, some treatment for minor infection and trauma, advice and alleviation of pain; and if further resources are available some emergency care. The rights and status of women were regarded as particularly decisive for furthering development. Governments were also made responsible for regulating any social or private health insurance schemes for clinical services outside the basic package, and for monitoring health provision and financing.

The World Bank was heavily criticised for the ideas promoted in this report, particularly those referring to user fees, structural adjustment, use of DALYs and privatisation (for example, Ruger, 2005: 68). As a consequence of such criticism, the World Bank's own Operations

Evaluation Development Department reviewed World Bank projects. It pointed to the narrow focus on capital investment, the focus on the immediate situation and the fragmented HNP portfolio. This has led to a shift away from basic health services to broader policy reforms, and the 1997 HNP Sector Strategy Paper (see also World Bank, 1997: 15; Ruger, 2005). As the 1997 Strategy further explains: "Recently, these observations led the bank to focus more on systemic reforms, both in the case of broad health systems/financing reforms and in the case of more targeted interventions" (World Bank, 1997: 15).

The 1997 HNP Sector Strategy Paper points out the important role of the World Bank in generating and diffusing knowledge, as well as in supporting projects financially. Two of the HNP objectives as formulated here are *enhancing the performance of health systems* and *securing sustainable health care financing*. In 2007, the World Bank formulated a revised strategy paper that reflects some changes with regard to the objectives in the HNP sector. The revised strategy paper appears a bit more cautious in the reasonable scope of engagement. While the 1997 strategy included the objectives to

> assist client countries to [...] enhance the performance of health care systems by promoting equitable access to preventive and curative health, nutrition, and population services that are affordable, effective, well managed, of good quality, and responsive to clients [and] secure sustainable health care financing by mobilizing adequate levels of resources, establishing broad-based risk pooling mechanisms, and maintaining effective control over public and private expenditure.
>
> (World Bank, 1997)

The later strategy said that among the World Bank's objectives was to increase assistance to countries related to their health care systems (World Bank, 2007: section 40), and "although focus on strengthening health systems is essential, this strengthening is seen as a crucial means for helping countries achieve HNP results rather than a policy objective in itself" (World Bank, 2007: section 36).

In summary, the World Development Report 1993 had proposed reducing government expenditure for anything other than basic health care and public health interventions. The concern was – and can still be seen in some of today's policy papers by World Bank staff

(Gwatkin et al., 2005; Yazbeck, 2006) – that scarce public spending could be wasted on rich people, who could also buy their health care to the detriment of the poor. As this only concerns the public-private distinction in terms of state/taxation versus out-of-pocket spending, the question of decentralisation (at the level of pooling) becomes obsolete. The 1997 strategy paper also marks a change in this regard: the focus shifted to risk-protection and pooling mechanisms (plus the mobilisation of additional resources). At the same time, it continues to state that essential health services should be financed publicly. (De)centralisation is still not an issue in the debate and the issue of user fees, which was an important element in earlier work and discussions, has almost disappeared. This more or less continues for the 2007 strategy paper. Here, however, it is mentioned that decentralisation in health financing is probably not useful; nevertheless, community financing could be a means to extending coverage.

Regulation

On regulation in general, the 2007 HNP strategy paper refers to the stewardship concept and term of the World Health Report 2000 (World Bank, 2007: sections 84, 90, and Annex L). Issues of governance and accountability were included as a new policy objective of the World Bank's work in HNP (World Bank, 2007: section 36). The issue at stake is seen as the adjustment of public policy to facilitate a viable public-private complementarity in health care provision and financing, to improve access to services for the poor and "to ensure effective regulation to enhance equity and efficiency" (World Bank, 2007: sections 59, 81).

The World Development Report 2004 on services makes the case for a certain level of cross-subsidies, either through social insurance or general taxation (World Bank, 2003: 146). The regulatory link between government and providers is summarised by this report as a monitoring of the benchmark performance of services; fostering of autonomous providers for clinical services; and the establishment of a strong monitoring function (World Bank, 2003: 149). The World Bank's new strategy further remarks that financial risk pooling is the "core function of health insurance mechanisms", and states:

> Participation in effective risk pooling is essential to ensure financial risk protection. It is also essential to avoid payment at the

moment of utilizing the services, which can deter people, especially the poor from seeking health care when sick or injured. Each society chooses a different way of pooling its people's financial risk to finance its health care system. Most high-income countries follow one of the two main models: the Bismarck model [...] or the Beveridge model [...] Improving financial protection in Bank client countries requires a substantial effort to increase participation in risk pooling.

(World Bank, 2007: Annex L)

These ideas of insurance models have also been addressed in "Health Financing Revisited: a Practitioner's Guide" (Gottret and Schieber, 2006), suggesting that "[v]oluntary and community-based financing schemes can serve as pilots for countries as they seek to expand the role of prepaid health coverage schemes".[24] The ideas about the system of financing do not include a clear model regarding the remuneration of providers.

On regulation, in summary, the World Development Report 1993 gives governments an important role in regulating private and social health insurance, in defining the benefit package according to cost-effectiveness criteria, and in other areas, such as giving particular attention to women's rights and status, and monitoring health provision and financing. This, again, sounds different in the 1997 strategy paper: here, the state is made responsible for securing equitable, universal access (combined with some targeting) to preventive and curative care; and for controlling public and private expenditure and provision. The regulatory role of the state should be strengthened, while for the other functions, private involvement should be increased. This is similar once more in the 2007 strategy paper. In contrast, the World Development Report 2004 was more explicit with regard to cross-subsidies through insurance or general taxation. Risk-pooling is now an important component of ideas on health financing (World Bank, 2007).

Universal health coverage

In Section 2.4, I showed a shift towards the concept and approach of UHC. The main World Bank papers just described are less specific about the benefit package, unless it is about particular health issues such as maternal health care or HIV/AIDS (see for example World

Bank, 2007). In recent years, however, the shift in attention to UHC has also had an effect on and been reflected in the World Bank. UHC, according to the World Bank's website, is about the following:

> All people aspire to receive quality, affordable health care. Universal health coverage (UHC) is about people having access to the health care they need without suffering financial hardship. UHC aims to achieve better health and development outcomes, help prevent people from falling into poverty due to illness, and give people the opportunity to lead healthier, more productive lives.[25]

In a joint paper on UHC, WHO and the World Bank stated: "UHC has been defined as a situation where all people who need health services (prevention, promotion, treatment, rehabilitation, and palliative) receive them, without undue financial hardship (World Health Report, 2010)" (WHO and World Bank, 2013: 2). That included three components: a comprehensive package of high-quality health services, provided on the basis of need; limited direct payments for health services; and universal coverage. UHC is particularly important with a view on the future development agenda, as expressed in that paper. The paper develops ideas about what matters for, and how to measure, UHC.

While concern about UHC brings the World Bank and WHO together, it needs to be taken into account that there is an important degree of contradiction in the World Bank's work and approach. This arises from the fact that another organisation within the World Bank Group, the IFC, for some years has been increasingly active in health issues and has developed its own health strategy. The following section examines this organisation.

International Finance Corporation (IFC)

The IFC's Articles of Agreement state that the purpose of the organisation is "to further economic development by encouraging the growth of productive private enterprise in member countries, particularly in the less developed areas, thus supplementing the activities of the International Bank for Reconstruction and Development" (article 1). As for the World Bank in general, this takes place with the intention of fighting poverty, follows a "country-by-country approach" and is "guided by our overreaching goals in the sector (to improve

health outcomes, to protect the population from the impoverish-
ing effects of ill health, and to enhance performance of health
services)."[26] However, the IFC is only concerned with private sector involvement. Its specific strategy for the health sector is set
out on its website, where it presents two further objectives for the
sector:

> The **business objective** aims to provide value-added financing to
> viable projects. The **development objective** seeks to ensure that
> our investments contribute to institutional and systemic capacity
> building and promote efficiency and innovation within the sector,
> while improving health security and expanding financial protec-
> tion against impoverishing effects of ill health. These objectives
> govern the way in which potential projects are screened and how
> they are monitored. Together with the analysis of global trends
> and IFC experience to date, they form the basis for our overall
> investment strategy.

Accordingly, the IFC's investments concentrate on the hospital sector, but are also expanding to non-hospital investments, including
private health insurance, pharmaceutical and medical devices and
health workers' education and training. It is further worth noting
that the IFC has both a profit goal and a development goal. Offi-
cially, the IFC "complements the work of the World Bank in public
sector reform, by focusing on the development of the private sector"
(Lethbridge, 2005: 207).

From an examination of the IFC Health Care Strategy,[27] it is evident
that the health policy approach of the IFC shows clear differences
to that of the World Bank as described above. Based on its general
purpose to support "open and competitive markets in developing
countries, support companies and other private sector partners, and
generate productive jobs and deliver basic services" (IFC Articles of
Agreement), the IFC sets out its health strategy as providing it with
the "opportunity to play a pioneer role" through supporting private
sector involvement via health project financing.

It is surprising – particularly considering the common understanding that prevails in World Bank documents – how the IFC describes
the situation of health care systems that support its role and responsibilities in the sector. The strategy argues that, so far, there has been

reliance only on the public sector, and that had not proved to be viable and sustainable. Other World Bank documents argue that there are private actors in place and that the health sector should be regulated in a way that meets the expectations of improving health. In contrast, the IFC explains:

> Global trends point to a significant and expanding role of the private sector as a partner with public health systems, particularly in the provision of health care. [...] The aim of much of the recent health care reforms in various countries has been to increase the role of the private sector as the provider (rather than the financier) of care, while complementing the activities of the public sector. The general argument is that these reforms can retain equity in the financing of health care, yet promote efficiency by introducing and encouraging competition.[28]

The strategy does not provide evidence for this view of the situation of health care systems, nor does it properly define them. Furthermore, there is no justification as to why the IFC nevertheless also attempts to enter the health insurance market with the aim of increasing private involvement. A further important omission is that the threat of fragmentation (when supporting single hospitals and so on) is not addressed at all.

What is provided by the IFC is, thus, not really a comprehensive health care system model, but a commitment to supporting the private sector, without it-being integrated into the activities of other global health actors (including the other World Bank Group organisations) with a more comprehensive view on the issue. Accordingly, the IFC's work does not feature any reflections about regulatory issues in health care systems.

Therefore, the IFC, concerned with supporting the private sector, has developed a health strategy on its own; by arguing that the other World Bank support for the public sector has not proved to be particularly successful. On the basis of its business objective, the IFC has increased its support to private providers and also attempts to intervene in health insurance arrangements. The IFC's strategy does not provide evidence for a comprehensive account of knowledge of or research into health care systems, but instead sticks with the simple idea of private sector support.

Overall, the World Bank (IBRD, IDA) has a long history of engagement in health, both in its lending and research activity, while the IFC engagement is recent, but ambitious. In the course of time, World Bank ideas have changed: more attention has been given to the health sector, particularly acknowledging that economic principles that might have worked in other policy fields are not necessarily translatable to health. This has included taking into account ideas from the WHO and also criticism from civil society organisations (Shaw, 2007). The World Bank is concerned about both equity and efficiency, while that approach is not easily to be found in IFC activity. The latter is understandable given the IFC's objective and focus and particularly its business objective; however, from the perspective of overall health care system policy, this approach does not meet the current state of knowledge about desirable health policy. The fact that World Bank and IFC staff have also jointly engaged in publishing on health (see Preker et al., 2007), does not appear to have changed the IFC's approach. As a consequence, the IFC's activities appear not only to be poorly contextualized with regard to the context of health care systems, but the World Bank Group's approach as a whole is uncoordinated.[29]

Dissemination Strategies

It needs to be taken into account that compared to other international organisations, the World Bank is particularly well equipped to disseminate its ideas. For example, it is able to run frequent courses on health care systems. What is actually being taught in the courses – at least judging from the course material and other material that can be obtained through the World Bank Institute's websites – follows many of the ideas just described. Roberts et al., for example, write[30]:

> In general we observed that to truly provide risk protection, a universal system based on ability to pay is required. It is no surprise, then, that middle- and upper-income countries mostly rely on social insurance or general revenue to finance their healthcare systems. As countries move up the development scale, social insurance is often especially attractive because the social contract implicit in such a system often improves tax compliance. [...]

In poor countries, household surveys reveal that even poor people pay substantial amounts out-of-pocket for care – [...]. To more effectively utilize these funds we believe community financing and other forms of decentralization have much to offer. [...]

Finally, we view with some trepidation the growth of private insurance in upper-middle-income nations.

(2008: 315ff.)

Finding other ways of directly engaging with governments is a particularly critical issue in the World Bank's work. The core of its work directed towards countries is aimed at giving different kinds of loans, which are given along with conditions. The World Bank has been heavily criticised for the use, and alarming effects, of these, on the one hand by civil society (for example, tribunals on the World Bank[3]) and on the other in academic literature (in the case of Uganda Macrae et al., 1996; also Koivusalo and Ollila, 1997 and Wogart, 2003). For the transition countries of Central and Eastern Europe, Radin (2003: 34)[32] interestingly argues that

[a]lthough the World Bank has been more aggressive in its participation of other social reforms such as the pension system in Poland, it has been comparatively shy in its assistance to the healthcare sector. [...] the first reason [...] lack of knowledge or internal conflict within the organization [...] IBRD chose not to get involved where success was not foreseeable.

Later in this book, it is argued that this hesitation in proposing clearly distinguishable models for health care systems (in contrast to pension models) is a typical feature of the global discourse on health care systems. At the same time, however, interventions in other fields, most importantly the general recommendation to cut public expenditures (including those in health) has in the past restricted the scope for the expansion of comprehensive health care systems (Koivusalo and Ollila, 1997; Wogart, 2003; McCoy, 2007; see also for example World Bank, 2008).

Disseminating ideas in academic communities is facilitated by the World Bank's organised networking. It has been discussed to what extent the World Bank uses the Global Development Network (GDN) in order to communicate ideas and strengthen its position as a "knowledge bank" (see also Stone, 2003; St Clair, 2006b).

Even in the case of the IFC, with obviously a limited attention on health issues, we see a "perfect" internet appearance, and its "voice" seems to be louder than its role and the scope of its health activities suggest. The IFC even organised an International Health Conference "Private Health Care in Emerging Markets – Evolution or Revolution?" on 18–20 April 2007, bringing together investors, specialists and financiers to explore the future of private health care and discuss business opportunities.[33] In the meantime, according to its own website the IFC is "[t]he world's largest multilateral investor in private health care [...] sectors in emerging markets".[34] On its role, the IFC website emphasises:

> As part of its new global agenda, IFC is leveraging its knowledge and understanding of private health care to work more closely with providers based in developed economies who are looking to expand their investments into under-served developing countries. Our strategy is to encourage and provide financing for the expansion of these global providers into new markets to build capacity and increase access to services. Developing country companies also benefit from global knowledge and expertise.[35]

At the same time, though, limiting the transformative power of the World Bank, the organisation continues to be automatically associated by many of its observers with specific sets of policy recommendations. This means that it is often judged and looked at through "neoliberal glasses", in the sense of the expectation that any idea uttered by the World Bank is neoliberal. This shapes the World Bank's potential to communicate particular ideas (which might be somewhat different from the alleged stereotype) in two ways. The IFC's increasing activities in the field that do not seem quite in line with the mainstream of current World Bank (IDA, IBRD) thinking support the concerns of critical outside observers. On the one hand, the World Bank's critical environment is sometimes somewhat resistant to acknowledging changes in ideas. On the other hand, national policymakers might have a stereotypical idea about what the World Bank wants to hear when applying for loans. Both forms limit the actual ability of the Bank to communicate (other than common neoliberal) ideas and cost, and to some extent limit credibility or trust in the institution – a mistrust that might not always be justified.

It is, however, also important to consider that World Bank staff working in different units, or on more or less theoretical issues, sometimes have different ideas, and not all of them are communicated in the same way. This means that those who are closely involved in on-the-ground activities might be more driven by standard neoliberal thinking than those involved with research into health care systems. Accordingly, while the World Bank is able to use a whole range of communication channels, this does not automatically mean that the messages the World Bank's intends to send out are properly taken up by outside observers and partners.

2.6   International Monetary Fund (IMF)

The International Monetary Fund (IMF) is commonly even more suspiciously observed than the World Bank. The IMF is the international organisation for international monetary cooperation – it "was created in 1945 to help promote the *health* of the world economy" (emphasis added).[36] But is the IMF also an international health policy actor? And if so, to what extent is this the case?

The primary purpose of the IMF is "to ensure the stability of the international monetary system – the system of exchange rates and international payments that enables countries (and their citizens) to buy goods and services from each other".[37] This is done, amongst other things, by providing advice to the member states; granting temporary financing to member countries to help them address balance of payment issues; and providing technical assistance and training.

Before the global and financial crisis of 2008, it was only low- and middle-income countries that sought help from the IMF, a situation that had forced the organisation to adjust its instruments, and to intensely collaborate with the World Bank to appropriately address the needs of these countries. At that time, even the very existence of the IMF was frequently questioned. For example, Martin Wolf in the *Financial Times*, 2006, said: "Let us be brutal: the IMF is on the brink not just of 'obscurity' as Mr. King (Governor, Bank of England) suggests but of irrelevance".[38] Other worries about the IMF in the mid-2000s concerned a budgetary crisis (Bello, 2006), conditionalities (Radelet, 2006) and – the most pressing issue in recent years – the representation of countries in IMF decision-making. However, it has not only been the observing civil society community that has been critical of the IMF's policies; the External Review Committee of the IMF has also criticised the IMF's role in low-income countries.[39]

Since the beginning of the global economic and financial crisis in 2008, the IMF has seen its largest period of upheaval since the 1990s (following the fall of the Berlin Wall); however, the criticism has continued as well, particularly its role in the recovery of Greek and Portuguese economies and its request for pro-cyclical economic policies, has been criticised (Bretton Woods Project, 2011). The concerns about the implications of IMF procedures in the health sector have remained the same.

The IMF's main business has always been macroeconomic and financial sector policies. However, advice on economic policy may easily overlap with issues also connected with the health sector, or at least have implications for choices and decisions about health policy. A study from the Center for Global Development Working Group on IMF Programs and Health Spending (Center for Global Development, 2007: viii f) argued that while many health policy issues go beyond the IMF's competence, "the content of IMF programs can have important indirect effects on the health sector, through size of overall spending and other influences", and concludes that "in several important ways, the IMF has often been too restrictive by ruling out potentially viable policy options without sufficient consideration" (Center for Global Development, 2007: x).

Even if the IMF might be tempted to overlook the impact of its activities on health, or think that related expertise should come from the World Bank, a paper by Heller and Hsiao – from more or less within the IMF – has been written with the hope of teaching IMF staff the basics of the health sector to provide them with some understanding of what they might be dealing with (Hsiao and Heller, 2007). From the outside, for example, Médecins Sans Frontières has criticised the IMF for encouraging countries to set limits on public spending, with detrimental effects for health care delivery (Médecins sans Frontières, 2007). The CGD's Working Group on IMF Programs and Health Expenditures comes to similar conclusions (Center for Global Development, 2007).

Reflecting on the usual fights between IFIs and UN social agencies, as described in other contributions to the global social policy literature, we can say that we see some elements of differences between the World Bank/IMF and WHO. Particularly in terms of the contents of ideas, the difference is more between the large majority of international organisations and the IFC in terms of ideas, and the IMF in terms of its conditionalities in particular countries (see also Kaasch, 2013; Deacon, 2014).

2.7   International Labour Organization: Long tradition but limited impact?

Introduction

The story, though, is not complete if we just contrast the IFIs with *one* "UN social agency" (namely the WHO as the one most relevant for this particular field of social policy). It is not only WHO that matters regarding health care systems. Given that health care systems have also been considered to being part of broader systems of social policy or the welfare state, the International Labour Organization (ILO) comes into focus. The organisation was established in 1919 as the UN agency concerned with the promotion of social justice and internationally recognised human and labour rights. It formulates international labour standards, amongst other things, in the fields of social security and occupational safety and health, including work on the expansion of welfare programmes. The ILO operates somewhat differently to other international organisations as it has a tripartite governance structure, with representatives of the government, organised labour and the business community of each member state who meet in the International Labour Conference (ILC) (see also Deacon, 2013).

The ILO's mandate in health is embedded in both its engagement in social security matters and a concern about occupational health and safety. It is specified in various documents, namely the Constitution of the ILO, the Declaration of Philadelphia, ILO Recommendations and Conventions (particularly the Medical Care ILO Recommendation No. 69 from 1944; the Social Security (Minimum Standards) Convention 1952 (No. 102) and the Medical Care and Sickness Benefits Convention 1969 (No. 130)), in the ILO's decent work concept, and in the New Consensus on Social Security. More concretely, the rationale for the ILO's engagement in health is based on the understanding that exclusion from social protection in health is a widespread and significant problem when it concerns, amongst other things, human rights and illness-inflected unemployment and disability. Thus, social protection in health is described as a key instrument in fighting poverty, addressing income security and improving access to health services, and also as contributing to the health-related MDGs.

The ILO's Social Protection Department (formerly Social Security Department) is particularly important. Its objectives are the enhancement of capacity of social security managers and the design and administration of sustainable social security schemes. The Global Campaign on Social Security and Coverage for All has served as a platform for the attainment of these objectives. Further, within the STEP (Strategies and Tools against Social Exclusion and Poverty) programme the extension of social protection coverage and reduction of poverty of workers in the informal sector has been pursued. In the STEP programme, the health sector was particularly focused upon when the extension of social security was being discussed. More recently, there has been work on designing a minimum package of social protection as a global social security floor (ILO Social Security Department, 2007, 2008).

Even though the ILO is not usually considered to be an important global health actor, this section shows that some ideas were formulated first by the ILO; and it was even proposed on occasion as *the* official organisation to deal with health insurance matters (Siddiqi, 1995). At the same time, the ILO's health care system ideas appear to have emerged in a somewhat different form to those of the organisations looked at so far. Health care systems are important as one element in systems of social protection, not genuinely as an institution responding to specific health needs.

Health care systems and the ILO: Workers or more?

Besides consideration of health in early general documents, namely the ILO Convention from 1919 and the Declaration of Philadelphia of 1944,[40] specifically on health, there have been early conventions, namely the Social Security (Minimum Standards) Convention 1952 (No. 102) and the Medical Care and Sickness Benefits Convention 1969 (No. 130). These still apply and are referred to in recent ILO documents (for example, International Labour Office, 2001). Ideas about health care systems, particularly with regard to forms of social health insurance, have also been developed in the World Labour Report 2000 (International Labour Office, 2000), Social Security: A New Consensus (International Labour Office, 2001) and, more recently, concepts emanating from the Global Campaign on Social Security and Coverage for All (ILO Social Security Department, 2007, 2008).

Originally, the context of dealing with health care systems has been strongly connected with the ILO's concern about workers. The link between this traditional focus of the ILO and health can be described as two-fold and has led to different streams of health-related work: on the one hand, there is health in the workplace (occupational health issues); on the other hand, and the focus here, health is a dimension of social security that shapes the lives of workers. Health is understood as a precondition to work, but also as a personal need, and the approach to social security in health focuses on health insurance (ILO Conventions 102 and 130). The World Labour Report 2000 further mentions the adverse effect of ill health on people's earning capacity, the financial risks of ill health and the rising overall cost of health care as important problems for the health sector (International Labour Office, 2000). The principles of health care systems are importantly connected to social justice, equity and targets for unemployment, poverty reduction and the promotion of common welfare, as can be seen in the ILO Convention from 1919 and the Declaration of Philadelphia of 1944 (see also International Labour Office, 2000; ILO Social Security Department, 2007, 2008). The strong focus on workers has been adjusted to global realities, such as significant numbers of people working in the informal sector. Deacon (2013: 27) explains: "while the so-called first-generation standards, [...], were only about social insurance, this had actually changed with the post-war adoption of Recommendation 67 and 69. These documents speak clearly about providing income security and medical care *to all*." The universal application is particularly evident in a recent paper from the ILO:

> To be meaningful, legal health coverage needs to result in effective access for all residents of a country, regardless of the financing subsystem to which they belong. However, this does not preclude national health policies from focusing temporarily on priority groups such as the most vulnerable when extending social

protection in health. Frequently, vulnerable population groups do not have equal access to necessary health care.

(Scheil-Adlung, 2014: 6)

Similar to the World Bank's approach, the ILO's accounts of health care systems are not particularly concerned about defining health care systems in a comprehensive way; they are more about establishing their role in order to achieve specific aims and principles. While the Alma-Ata Declaration is often called the first document to give the responsibility for health care explicitly to the state (Koivusalo and Ollila, 1997; Kickbusch, 2000), it is interesting to see that the Medical Care Recommendation of 1944 already

> generally recognised [...] that the State has the overall responsibility for creating a medical care service for all persons, whether or not they are gainfully employed, with a view to: a) restoring health (providing curative care), and b) protecting and improving health (providing preventive care).
>
> (ILO and ISSA, 1997: 6; see also International Labour Office, 2001: section 2; International Labour Office, 2005: fourth item on the agenda)

Similarly, the World Labour Report 2000, amongst other things, was intended to "show [...] how governments can work to guarantee access for all to health care and protect individuals from the detrimental effects of poor health on income security".[41]

Provision

At the same time, however, the ILO's traditional focus on workers and concepts of processes for extending *coverage* (instead of comprehensive models of coverage of all) as in the ILO Convention 102 on Social Security (Minimal Standards) results in an astonishing set of requirements. Namely, it

> does not require that the full range of health care is available to the whole population, indeed the Convention's requirements are satisfied with 50 per cent of employees, 20 per cent of the economically active population, or 50 per cent of residents
>
> (ILO and ISSA, 1997: 6)

In later accounts (International Labour Office, 2001), the proposed degree of coverage is not entirely clear either: is it about universal coverage or just social insurance for workers (and their dependents)? The 1952 Convention also says that insurance should cover "a substantial part of the persons whose earnings do not exceed those of the skilled manual male employee" (Article 6). However, Article 9 talks about prescribed classes of employees and their families. The convention of 1969 goes further in defining the groups to be included as a large part of the economically active population and residents in general. As far as people are part of an insurance scheme, health care is to be provided according to need ("[...] in respect of a condition requiring medical care of a preventive or curative nature [...]", Article 7). Also, the new consensus on social security reaffirms:

> Social security covers health care [...] It is not always necessary, nor even in some cases feasible, to have the same range of social security provision for all categories of people. However, social security systems evolve over time and can become more comprehensive in regard to categories of people and range of provisions as national circumstances permit. Where there is limited capacity to finance social security, either from general tax revenues or contributions – and particularly where there is no employer to pay a share of the contribution – priority should be given in the first instance to needs which are most pressing in the view of the groups concerned.
>
> (ILO, 2001: 4)

Following work has explicitly focused on extending social security, including health care, for all (ILO Social Security Department, 2007, 2008). Particularly interesting in this respect is the paper by Xenia Scheil-Adlung (2014). Related to the development of the social protection floor (SPF) initiative (for a detailed account of its background and meaning see Deacon, 2013), this social protection policy paper on universal health protection "is intended to inform about available policy options for developing and improving coverage and effective access to health care. [...] The policy options discussed focus on ensuring the human rights to social security and health and on the rights-based approaches underpinning the need for equity and poverty alleviation" (Scheil-Adlung, 2014: v). The paper explains that, as part of Recommendation No 202, health protection is considered as feasible at any level of GDP, including an element of prevention, "an investment in people rather than a tool to redistribute income" and a genuinely global issue (p. 3). On the basis of that, the SPFs aim at introducing universal in-kind benefits and basic income (p. 3). Social protection in health is defined, referring to the World Social Security Report 2010/2011 as "a series of public or publicly organized and mandated private measures against social distress and economic loss caused by the reduction of productivity, stoppage or reduction of earnings or necessary treatment that can result from ill health" (ILO, 2010: 35). The related system should be needs-based and aim at "achieving universal coverage" (Scheil-Adlung, 2014: 6).

Financing

Explicitly, the ILO documents do not say much about the *provision* function and focus instead on health *financing* options. The World Labour Report 2000 names three financing mechanisms – taxation, insurance and non-insurance funding systems – and explains that most countries use a combination of the three (International Labour Office, 2000: 83). Critical about decentralised financing systems, the report is very much in favour of insurance systems, particularly social health insurance. This is because they make it possible to ensure a right to a defined benefit package and access to care depending on need. It is not only the system as such, but also the options it offers related to processes of decision-making:

> Social health insurance revenues are managed independently and separately from general government revenue by autonomous institutions. These institutions are generally governed by tripartite or bipartite governing bodies composed of representatives of those who finance the health insurance scheme (i.e. workers, employees and – if applicable – governments).
>
> (International Labour Office, 2000: 85)

Considerable space is given to discussing the option of micro-insurance schemes as "a complementary strategy to improve equity of access to health care for the excluded" (International Labour Office, 2000: 87–88). Also, this mechanism is process-related and includes the idea of community members participating in decisions about the scheme. Such micro-insurance schemes "are not, however, designed to become the main pillar of a country's health financing system" (International Labour Office, 2000: 87, 202ff.). Discussions at the 89th ILC in 2001 provide evidence for some disagreement between the workers' and the employers' parties within the ILO. The Worker Vice-Chairperson considered several options regarding the extension to a universal health care system, with micro-insurance schemes contributing only in a limited way. However, the Employer Vice-Chair rather saw micro-insurance as a successful option per se and warned against "placing an extra financial burden on employers and workers in the formal sector to finance benefits for the informal sector" (International Labour Office, 2001: 2–3). Community-based social protection schemes, for example models of micro-insurance, have been worked out and tested in the STEP programme. This has, for instance, included the development of study guides for micro-insurance schemes (ILO STEP, 2005).

The World Labour Report 2000 also discusses the option of user fees for the financing of health care systems, but does not support them owing to their regressive character and their uneven effects on access to and utilisation of health services, amongst other things (International Labour Office, 2000: 91ff.). There is no particular benefit package defined; rather the different kinds of care (for example, general practitioner care, specialist care) and decisions about essential pharmaceuticals are left to the medical profession. Cost-sharing (out-of-pocket contributions) is considered possible. Revenue collection should happen through insurance contributions or taxation. The contributions should be affordable for poorer people (International Labour Office, 2000).

Following the new consensus on social security, the Global Campaign on Social Security and Coverage for All was launched. As part of that, the most recent ILO attempt to conceptualise social security, including health care, has taken the shape in the concept of a social protection floor (for reference to a "Global Social Floor or Global Socio-economic Floor", see World Commission on the Social Dimension of Globalization (2004). The role of the state, in general, is described as "facilitator and promoter" (ILO Social Security Department, 2007: 27), and as sharing responsibilities for defining the functions and responsibilities for each subsystem of the health care system, including the development of a legal framework and ensuring adequate funding and services. The idea is to provide for a "base of social and economic rights that are outside the realm of social security" (ILO Social Security Department, 2008: 2). This basic set of guarantees includes, amongst other things, that "all citizens have access to basic/essential health care benefits through pluralistic delivery mechanisms where the state accepts the general responsibility for ensuring adequacy of the delivering system and its financing" (ILO Social Security Department, 2008: 2). The basic social transfers may be in cash or in kind and it is up to countries how to realise them, as they are "formulated as a set of guarantees rather than a set of defined benefits" (ILO Social Security Department, 2008: 3). Most likely, these guarantees would be financed through general taxation and, while integrated into a country's social security system, would be provided in the form of social assistance.

Regarding financing, the aforementioned paper by Scheil-Adlung states that it is not about a particular system, but key is a focus on the one hand on solidarity and sufficient income generation for the health care system while on the other "affordability and financial protection in addition to availability of quality services" (Scheil-Adlung, 2014: 6) is important – meaning no out-of-pocket payments. That should lead to equity in access to health care. Furthermore, "[i]nvestments in health through social protection are justified by human rights" (Scheil-Adlung, 2014: 11). In order to achieve that, the ILO Social Protection Floor Recommendation was proposed as a "guideline for achieving sustainable universal coverage in health" (p. 36).

Regulation

In that context, social health protection is defined as "a series of public or publicly mandated private measures against social distress and economic loss caused by the reduction of productivity, stoppage or reduction of earning or the cost of necessary treatment that can result from ill health" and it is "founded on burden sharing, risk pooling, empowerment and participation" (ILO Social Security Department, 2007: 3). The approach is to recognise all existing forms of social protection within a country or context. Accordingly, a discussion of different options for financing and organising health care systems follows. Further, policymakers are advised on ways to realise universal and equitable access, financial protection in health, and efficient and effective health care provision (ILO Social Security Department, 2007: 3). It is proposed:

> First, taking stock of all existing financing mechanisms
>   in a given country;
> Next, assessing the remaining access deficits, and
> Last, developing a coverage plan which fills gaps in an
>   efficient and effective way.
>
> (ILO Social Security Department, 2007: 27)

Far from providing a list of services that should form part of the benefit package, the ideas about the package have somewhat departed from a process-oriented to a substantial recommendation:

> The ILO advocates that benefit packages [...] should be defined with a view to maintaining, restoring and improving health, the ability to work and meet personal health-care needs. Key criteria for establishing benefit packages include the structure and volume of the burden of disease, the effectiveness of interventions, the demand and the capacity to pay.
>
> (ILO Social Security Department, 2007: 13)

However, this should (still) involve social partners and social dialogue in policy processes and governance schemes (ILO Social Security Department, 2007: 27–28, 37–38). The medical profession is also considered to be important in this process.

The paper provides a route to develop a comprehensive plan and strategy for the achievement of universal coverage that includes the development of a national health budget to assess the financial status and development of the health care system (ILO Social Security Department, 2007: 29). Concerning the governance of health care systems, with a particular view on financing, it says:

> In order to fulfil the criteria of good governance, the financial and administrative separation of health insurance funds from Ministries of Health and Labour is essential. Generally, revenues earmarked for social health protection should be separated from government budgets and it should be ensured that contributions

are used only for health-care benefits and administration of the scheme [...]

(ILO Social Security Department, 2007: 39)

It recommends decentralisation or organisational units, and strategic purchasing (ILO Social Security Department, 2007: 39).

The World Social Security Report 2010/2011 emphasises the role of legal universal coverage and effective access to health services. Essential benefit packages are supposed to run along the lines of nationally and internationally agreed objectives (for example, MDGs). It is further important that "ill health does not lead to catastrophic loss of income and impoverishment" (ILO, 2010: 36). As in many other accounts, it is "[p]re-payment and pooling [considered to] institutionalize [...] solidarity between the rich and the less well-off, and between the healthy and the sick" (ILO, 2010: 39) which can be reached in different ways, including public schemes, social insurance schemes, private insurance and community-based schemes (pp. 3–40).

Overall, it could be said that coming from a twin-streamed approach to health (health and safety at the workplace, and health as an element of social security), recent ILO work is evolving to embrace a concept of social security with social assistance (social health protection) while the workplace issue, of course, continues as well. The ILO was traditionally concerned about access to care; it has been ambiguous, though, about whether the concern was exclusively for workers and their dependents or for universal access including all citizens or inhabitants of a country.

Much emphasis has been on insurance systems, particularly social health insurance, which has been expected to ensure a right to a defined benefit package and access to care depending on need. The process of defining the benefit package has been linked to the ILO's tripartite governing and decision-making structure. Until recently, when it concerned the extension of coverage, the focus has been on micro-insurance schemes. Most recent ideas coming from the ILO, however, have concerned the introduction of the concept of social protection floors. This takes up the idea of the need for all people to be covered by a certain level of health care as a set of basic guarantees, financed through general taxation and integrated into a country's social security system (thus a form of social assistance). Accordingly, the ILO concept has evolved to accommodate other than primarily work-focused social security to elements of poverty reduction and social assistance.

Dissemination

Among the strategies that the ILO uses to strengthen its position as a global social policy actor is "[p]olicy advocacy and national and international partnerships with international organizations, international and regional banks, development agencies, and stakeholders, such as employees' and employers' organizations".[42] This has, for example, included encouraging "Show and Tell seminars" between different international organisations (Deacon, 2007: 67–68; see also O'Brien, 2008: 132); but more importantly the building of alliances to realise the global social protection floor, including with the World Bank (see Deacon, 2013). However, while many of the ILO's activities on health are very limited because few staff work on the issue, it is the global "health" organisation with perhaps the most expertise in social security systems, including health, which is able to facilitate international law in the field of health care systems. Suboptimal use of its website further constrains the communication of ideas and the visibility of work undertaken.

With a particular focus on one health financing model, the ILO, the German Enterprise for Technical Cooperation (GTZ)[43] and the WHO collaborated on developing and communicating ideas about social health insurance within the Consortium on Social Health Protection in Developing Countries.[44] The basic ideas to be found on the Consortium's website and in the Berlin Recommendations of Action (ILO et al., 2005) are the following: with a focus on poor countries, the context is described as a situation of very limited access to health services for poor people and catastrophic health expenditure. The basic principles or aims to be achieved are thus universality, equity and solidarity within sustainable systems of social (health) protection. Health (security) is considered as a human right, and the question is accordingly about universal access to effective and affordable health care (that is, preventive, curative and rehabilitative health interventions) (ILO et al., 2005: 3). Similarly to the ILO concepts above, the key to approaching this problem is a country's financing system (ILO et al., 2005: 4).

Furthermore the recommendations suggest that extending social protection in health can be done through various forms of taxation, insurance and mixed systems. The critical issue, however, is that of enhanced risk-sharing and risk-pooling, thus increasing the share of prepayment related to out-of-pocket payments. Ideally, this includes subsidies and cross-subsidies between risk pools. For social health insurance schemes, it is particularly stressed that they should also be based on principles of responsibility and participatory governance by the social partners and the insured; and, thus, regulation needs to be based on social dialogue.

Building up social protection in health should be part of a comprehensive strategy of health sector reform, should come with an increase in the level of health spending (including external money in low-income countries) and take into account the broader determinants of ill health, such as social exclusion. A mix of financing mechanisms is favoured, arguing:

> Combining contribution-based financing with tax-financed subsidies enables the coverage of population groups or specific epidemiological necessities. A mix of financing methods could share the burden of health care expenditures among a broader tax base while also promoting greater potential for cross-subsidy by having contributors and non-contributors in the same pool.
>
> (ILO et al., 2005: 5–6)

It is stressed that the route to universal coverage will be a long road and a complex one. The state is given an important role in the facilitation, promotion and extension of health protection, including regulating high-quality and low-cost (efficient) health care provision, including both public and private providers.

> Health care providers also need to be acquainted with the principles of modern health care purchasing arrangements, including the procedures of accreditation, contracting and payment mechanisms' advantages and limits within a third party payment agreement.
>
> (ILO et al., 2005: 10)

Concluding, the approach is based on the notion of health as a human right and strives to realise access for all to effective and affordable health care. The Consortium focuses on the financing dimension, promoting social health insurance for enhanced risk-sharing and risk-pooling. This includes elements of both the WHO and the ILO approaches.

2.8 Inter-actor relationships and health systems within the UN system

The previous sections about the different international organisations that function as global health actors – within the UN system – have revealed a number of issues. In this final section, the chapter's main insights will be taken up again and discussed within a context of a system of global health governance, understood as the respective relationships between these actors. Historically, it is interesting to see how the original struggle between the ILO and WHO about the actor which held the most legitimate position from which to speak about health care systems has shifted to one between the WHO and the World Bank. In a global health policy environment characterised by a number of actors involved in global social policy and in particular policy models for national health care systems, multiple vertical health initiatives and repetitive announcements about the importance of strengthening health care systems, the ILO tries to present and establish itself as a particularly important international organisation that is able to perform proper social and health budgeting in order to bring together external and internal financing in one system, as for example through social health insurance (SHI) models. This extends the concept of bipolar, competing actors or actor coalitions to one of fluctuating, multi-polar constellations that consider varying and multiple positions at different points in time. The struggles over positions are only partly about the content of policy models or prescriptions, but also to a large extent concern questions of legitimacy and acceptance (by member states and other international organisations).

In addition, we can observe contestation and collaboration between actors at the same point in time. The simultaneity of collaborative and rival interaction between these organisations is explained by distinguishing discourses at different levels of abstraction. For example, it is shown that the organisations' positions on health care systems as a whole are either quite similar or too vague to be easily discerned. At the same time, a number of global health discourses are about particular functions or mechanisms of health care systems, and they have been controversial; examples are the discourses on user fees and the privatisation of health provision.

This means that, for instance, while the World Bank itself does not describe its role in health and its expanding activities as concurrent with that of the WHO, literature on global health governance is rather critical about these activities and the position of the World Bank as the most powerful global health actor (Koivusalo and Ollila, 1997: 25; Kickbusch, 2000). However, apart from this question about the most powerful global health actor, the scene has also always been marked by collaboration, and ideas from one organisation are featured in the work of the other. For example, the World Bank's World Development Report 1993 Investing in Health has, on the one hand, been interpreted as the World Bank challenging the WHO's position (Koivusalo and Ollila, 1997: 30–31); but, on the other hand, Kickbusch (2000: 982) states that "[p]aradoxically the World Bank's interest in health went back to WHO's approach to the World Bank and the 1993 Investment in Health Report was the long term outcome of a meeting between WHO Director General Halfdan Mahler and the President of the World Bank MacNamara".

Another example would be the World Health Report 2000, which forms an important component of World Bank teaching material, and which is frequently quoted concerning basic definitions in World Bank work and statements.[45] An important objective of the World Bank Institute courses is, however, how to analyse and understand a problem and look for solutions, rather than exploring a particularly narrow policy idea or communicating concrete recommendations (Roberts et al., 2008). It is about analytical and practical tools, and the element of exchange between participants is an important component of the courses.

3
The OECD and the WTO: Outside the UN but Increasingly Important?

3.1 Introduction

Apart from the international organisations within the UN system, at least two other important and powerful international organisations need to be considered with regard to their influence on health care systems. This chapter first turns to the role of the Organisation for Economic Co-operation and Development (OECD); and then discusses the potential impact on health care systems that the World Trade Organization (WTO) exerts by facilitating trade agreements.

3.2 Organisation for Economic Co-operation and Development: Convincing advice by staying "neutral"?

Introduction

Traditionally, the OECD has strong links to the European region regarding history and member states, as it grew out of the Organisation for European Economic Co-operation (OEEC) of 1947 to coordinate the Marshall Plan for the reconstruction of Europe after the Second World War (OECD, 2005: 9). Currently, the OECD has 34 member states, many of them high-income countries. The OECD also, to some extent, relates to transition and developing countries that do not form part of the organisation (through its Development Center, and more indirectly through the Development Assistance Committee (DAC)). The organisation describes itself as "a unique forum where the governments of [...] market economies work together to address the economic, social and governance challenges of globalisation as well as to exploit its opportunities", and as providing "a setting where governments can compare policy experiences, seek answers to common problems, identify good practice and co-ordinate domestic and international policies [...] [and] where peer pressure can act as a powerful incentive to improve policy and implement 'soft law' " (OECD, 2005: 7).

In organisational terms, the OECD secretariat is responsible for producing information and analysis for the member states' governments. It collects data, monitors trends, analyses economic developments and researches social changes or evolving patterns in such fields as trade, technology and taxation (OECD, 2005: 7). In the field of health, related work is done within various directorates (in this context most importantly the Health Division in the Directorate for Employment, Labour and Social Affairs (DELSA)), coordinated by an Intra-Directorate Coordination Group for Health.[1]

A justification for the OECD's concern and activities in health issues can be derived from its general mission to improve the economic and social policies of its member states. However, the actual justification frequently provided by the OECD is that the background and focus of the OECD's engagement in health policy issues is down to an explicit demand from its member states for specific activities and engagement in health policies (for example, OECD, 2004b).

The OECD's engagement in the field of health has grown out of its statistical work. A first report specifically on health was Public Expenditure on Health (OECD, 1977). This report was part of a broader project about issues of resource allocation and government expenditure, undertaken by a working party to deal with questions of economic growth within the Economics Policy Committee. Its main interest was not health policy as such, but the expansion of the public sector. From the 1980s onwards, health has been approached under the social policy work of the OECD, beginning with a report on the Financing and Delivery of Health Care (OECD, 1987) and in the 1990s with a focus on health care reforms (OECD, 1992, 1993a, 1993b, 1994, 1995, 1996). While all this work had come with a strong emphasis on quantitative data and statistical concerns, particularly since the beginning of the 21st century, the OECD has expanded its health activities also to include more qualitative analytical work, as well as having begun peer reviews of the performance of single member state's health care systems. With the launch of the OECD Health

Project (from 2001) that part of the OECD's health work has increased significantly. The OECD Health Project concluded in 2004, releasing a final report (OECD, 2004b) as well as a number of other reports on the specific research topics undertaken as part of the Project (see for example the one on private health insurance discussed below, OECD, 2004a). Owing to the success of the OECD Health Project, the health policy-related work has been continued and even expanded.

Institutionally, this increased attention on health issues is reflected through the OECD Health Committee (earlier the Group on Health) directing the OECD work on health and advising the Council on appropriate priorities; in the creation of a new Division on Health within DELSA; and the comparably high number of staff working on health issues. At the same time other Directorates, namely that for Financial and Enterprise Affairs and also that for Fiscal Affairs, touch on the domain of health policy. Also, the Economic Development and Review Committee (EDRC) increasingly integrates social and health policy indicators and reasoning in the Economic Surveys.

Thus, while so far rather marginally considered in global health literature, the OECD has developed as an increasingly important global health actor. The strengthening of the OECD's position can be regarded as a consequence of the failed attempt by the WHO to rank health care systems (see also Chapter 2, section 4). Further, its ideas may go well beyond influencing its member states' thinking about health care systems (Deacon and Kaasch, 2008).

OECD ideas about health care systems

As to the context of health care systems, OECD publications are characterised by an understanding of health care as an important social service and, at the same time, an important economic factor (for example, OECD, 1987, 2004a). However, taking a historical look at the publications shows that it was some time before the current balanced socio-economic view was reached. Earlier publications seemed to have struggled somewhat with understanding health policy as something that cannot be captured only with economic thinking (see for example OECD, 1992: 14–15). It is only publications since around the year 2000 that treat health care with a more balanced, socio-economic approach; a typical statement being that health is both a major economic factor *and* an important element of social cohesion (OECD, 2000, 2004a).

The portfolio of OECD health work approaches the topic of health care systems in a broad and interdisciplinary way. However, while statistical work has been primarily directed to health care systems as a whole, the analytical work is characterised by a careful selection of specific health policy issues or topics that are identified as of particular interest to, or requested by, OECD member states. It includes issues around the organisation and performance of health care systems and is based on this broader statistical work.[2] The focus is mainly on OECD member states, but as part of its outreach work, the organisation also addresses other countries.

The basic (common) objectives, or principles, of health care systems identified by the OECD can be summarised as follows: accessible health care (for all citizens; adequate and equal), high-quality health care, (macro- and micro-) economic efficiency (in use and provision); and redistributional and income-protection functions are frequently listed (OECD, 1987, 1992, 1994, 2004a). The 1992 report further includes freedom of choice for consumers and appropriate autonomy of providers (OECD, 1992). These objectives, according to the publications, may vary between countries depending on their relative importance or rank.

The OECD approaches health care systems through their characteristic stories and problems, less by how they are defined. The general "health care system story" as described in OECD publications is that of a rapid growth of health care systems in OECD countries after 1945, followed by a relatively stable phase until the 1970s and 1980s, when many countries encountered for the first time financial constraints regarding health care. While the earlier reforms had focused on universal access and extending rights to health, the reforms of the 1970s and 1980s attended to tightening budgets. In this context, it became clear that health care delivery was inefficient. The OECD identifies remarkable changes in the situation and reform of health care systems in its member states since the mid-1990s. The general concern in related debates and reforms is a search for "strategies to enhance the effectiveness and responsiveness of health systems" (OECD, 1994: Foreword) connected to *efficiency* criteria (see for example OECD, 1987, 1992, 1994).

An important characteristic of the OECD's health approach, underlying its typical focus on comparison and mutual learning, is the identification of similarities, common challenges and problems of different health care systems. Accordingly, besides the "common story" as told above, there are also common characteristics, problems and solutions. The common problems frequently listed are, amongst others, the rising costs because of new medical technology; ageing populations and demographic change; increased utilisation of services (while also taking into account a certain degree of under-utilisation by some groups in the population); inappropriate use of services; the inadequacy of care, the lack of responsiveness; waiting times; biological, cultural and social factors; rising expectations; inappropriate incentives for providers, unsuitable organisational and management structures, poorly designed regulation mechanisms; gaps in information about effectiveness and costs (OECD, 1987, 1992, 1994, 2004a). The final report of the OECD Health Project adds that there are significant shortcomings in the *quality* of care (OECD, 2004b).

This balanced health approach that is – in addition – very much concerned not to openly and directly blame any member state, makes it very difficult (if not wrong) to identify a specific "health care system model" favoured by the OECD. However, there are still some points to make: earlier OECD publications were more willing to propose or express their preference for specific arrangements, such as the Health Maintenance Organisations (HMOs) and prospective reimbursement systems (OECD, 1987); or the public contract model,[3] said to be best suited for combining the strengths of public and private health care (OECD, 1992).

The 1992 report further describes managed markets as the most successful ones. However, this publication was a comparison of seven OECD countries – and thus the conclusions were based on these seven health care systems. Two years later, another study followed that compared the remaining 17 OECD member states, which partly altered these findings, concluding that there seems to be no relationship between successful cost containment and the organisation of health services (OECD, 1994). In contrast, the 2004 final report of the OECD Health Project does not favour any specific model or intervention but is characterised throughout by discussing advantages and drawbacks of different models. If there is a general recommendation, it is the call for more and better data. Tackling the lack of data issue, the OECD has its OECD Survey on Health Systems Characteristics.[4] Furthermore, a new report on health care system performance makes recommendations for addressing geographical variations in health care (OECD, 2014).

The functions of health care systems

The OECD publications on health care systems show a shift in the main focus between different health care system functions. Problems and possible solutions (reform options) in very early health work (OECD, 1977) concentrated on the financing function. The 1987 report paved the way for changes in the publications of the 1990s, when the belief was expressed that reforms and attempts to tackle health sector problems were mostly connected to provision: the need for more quality assurance and for better information on health outcomes and costs (OECD, 1992: 141). More recent OECD health publications are characterised by a tendency to see regulation as the main function that is crucial for any change. This change regarding health care system functions, however, is not to be understood as absolute or mutually exclusive. Owing to the OECD's careful approach to health care systems and its focus on particular issues connected to health care systems, some of the sub-functions of health care systems do not seem to be addressed, such as the remuneration of providers and benefit packages.

Accordingly, the OECD's approach in relation to health care systems is characterised by identifying a common story, common problems and common objectives for all OECD health care systems, and, from that, building the basis for mutual policy learning in how to approach common health policy problems and reform constraints. The more recent analyses are driven by a balanced socio-economic perspective, and, while there is no one model identified that is favoured by the secretariat, there are some characteristics of the OECD health approach. Among these are a very careful handling of policy recommendations, except for the general call for more and better data; an understanding of health care systems as consisting of different functions that can be driven by different public-private mixes; and a shift in functions that are most likely to make a change when reformed (financing to provision to regulation).

Dissemination

To the outside, the OECD has been best known for its data; for providing a reliable and trustworthy source of information for other international organisations, national policy makers, academics and others. Datasets include those produced for the Health Quality

Indicators Project, the System of National Health Accounts and the OECD Health Data.

Developing and disseminating such ideas, the OECD hosted a number of conferences focusing on health issues, including a conference in Canada in November 2001 discussing health care system performance with health care policymakers, managers, practitioners and experts as participants.[5] More importantly, in concluding its "Health Project", the OECD convened a meeting of OECD Health Ministers,[6] presenting the results of its work, providing a platform to discuss health issues and being given the mandate to conduct further work on a number of specified health issues. This event thus had multiple functions in terms of providing information from the perspective of the OECD; it was a platform for discussion among policymakers; and it also served the purpose of renewing the organisation's mandate on health care system issues.

In order to enhance its communication channels, the OECD strongly seeks to make links with academia, such as the Brookings Institutions. The organisation is engaged in joining and building epistemic communities to help its ideas travel (Deacon and Kaasch, 2008).[7]

A comprehensive report about the Health Project and related activities was published (OECD, 2004b), and a number of other publications have been released that also tackle health care systems (for example, Or, 2002a; Docteur and Oxley, 2003; OECD, 2004a). While some of these publications explain something about the OECD's activities in health, they can best be classified as research publications. In addition, and regarding its interaction with single member states, the OECD has started a series of health care system assessments on request (for example, on Switzerland, OECD and WHO, 2006). More readily taken up by policymakers and the public are the OECD's Economic Surveys of countries. These, however, increasingly include social and health issues, and collaboration between the OECD's departments is growing. Thus qualified recommendations on health care systems can be expected also to be transmitted through the release of such reports (see Deacon and Kaasch, 2008).

Conclusions

Overall, the OECD's health work is characterised by even-handed, high-quality indicators and analytical publications; and some exchange between national policymakers has taken place through the OECD. Initial country assessments of health care systems have been released, with all such work carefully balanced so as not to become a "naming and shaming" exercise, as has been character-istic for other policy fields, such as education. However, as OECD health work is still evolving, it is difficult to forecast its future role (for related discussions see Mahon and McBride, 2008a; Martens and Jakobi, 2010).

Before considering other organisations, one further remark is nec-essary. What has been described so far applies first and foremost to OECD member states, which are a fairly small group of high-income countries. However, it was noted earlier that the OECD also carries out outreach work with non-member states. Importantly, this work does not appear to be as even-handed and careful as for member states, although a much more detailed analysis would be needed to understand the OECD's role in this respect (Kaasch, 2010). What is interesting, however, is that the MDGs, including those on health, originated from the OECD's DAC and thus, to some extent, have been shaped by ideas developed within the OECD secretariat (Deacon and Kaasch, 2008). This implies that the OECD may have more signifi-cant impact on development policies than its membership suggests. Apart from specific advice given to non-OECD member states, there may also be more indirect impacts on health care systems of countries that receive development aid, as advised by the OECD with regard to appropriate targets or goals.

3.3   World Trade Organization: Significant or speculative impact on health care systems?

While even less obviously a "health actor" than many of the organ-isations already discussed, a number of authors have pointed to the role and potential impact of the WTO with regard to national health care systems (for example, Koivusalo, 1999, 2003c; Holden, 2005). The possible implications for the field of social and health policy resulting from the WTO's activities are suspected to emerge from the "basic underlying philosophy of the WTO [...] that open markets, non-discrimination, and global competition in international trade are conducive to the national welfare of all countries" (Koivusalo, 1999: 15),[8] and "in general health [...] impacts are considered in the

WTO mostly as consequence of economic growth which is presented as yielding cheaper consumer products, [and] health technology improvements [...]" (Koivusalo, 1999: 15). Thus, while potentially influencing national health policy and having been described as "a new potential forum for many labour, environmental and health related matters" (Koivusalo, 2003c: 2), the agreements of the WTO, namely the Agreement on Trade-related Aspects of Intellectual Property Rights (TRIPS) and the General Agreement on Trade in Services (GATS), as well as the pronouncements of this international organisation, cannot be interpreted as contributing ideas about *best* health care systems. Instead, the problem is said to be in the WTO's "focus on health care as an industry [that] may easily lure attention away from the fundamental functions of a health care system" (Koivusalo, 2003c: 7).

The literature about the WTO as a global actor within the field of health policy mainly focuses on the implications of the two WTO agreements – TRIPS (for example, Koivusalo, 1999) and GATS (for example, Sexton, 2001; Woodward, 2005; Yeates, 2005) – for national health (and social) policy. While discussing the potential dangers that such trade agreements might have for national health policies, both streams of argumentation have been described as being "largely speculative in nature" (Woodward, 2005: 515). Critics fear that international agreements on trade "may in practice also effectively limit government abilities to impose regulatory measures" (Koivusalo, 1999: 37; see also Timmermans, 2004) and that it will lead "towards less effective, costlier and inequitable health systems development" (Koivusalo, 1999: 38). Further, there is concern that the hidden dangers of making commitments regarding health services, such as what a certain regulation actually means for the health sector, would not be obvious at the moment of signing the agreement (Koivusalo, 1999: 39; Timmermans, 2004: 454), and could be very difficult to change later (Sexton, 2001; Woodward, 2005). It is also feared that commitments in the field of health services could be enforced by trade sanctions (Koivusalo, 1999: 18; Sexton, 2001: 5). The critics of WTO politics in relation to social or health policies also point to the risks of WTO agreements regarding public policies more generally. Koivusalo (1999: 18), calling this problem "trade-creep", argues that "WTO policies may have 'creeping impacts' in public policies, which cannot be dealt with solely in the context of trade interests of countries, and may lead to systematic adverse incentives and impacts upon health and social policies." It is also acknowledged that so far, for example, GATS has not been an important driver of privatising health services, even though such services are listed there as potentially open to competition; and that the WTO accepts governments' hesitation to commercialise hospitals (Sexton, 2001: 18; Vanduzer, 2005: 189).

More concretely on GATS, this agreement (in effect since 1995) has different parts: a framework agreement containing the general rules and disciplines; and the national "schedules" (individual countries list their specific commitments). It defines rules for international trade in practically all services, without a definition of services as such (Sexton, 2001: 4). For the health service sector, there are four subsectors: medical and dental services; nursing and midwifery; hospital services; and other health services. GATS comprises four modes, namely cross-border provision of services (for the field of health, for example, telemedicine), cross-border movement of consumers (for example, cross-border movement of patients to receive health services), commercial presence of providers (for example, foreign ownership of health facilities) and cross-border movement of providers (for example, temporary migration of health professionals).

Woodward (2005: 515) distinguishes two streams of literature concerning GATS and the trade in health services: a *trade* faction emphasising the developmental chances arising through trade without really looking at health care systems, and the *health care system* faction discussing the dangers to health care systems. Still, even the critics admit that – up to now – the implications of GATS have been limited, as those services that are primarily provided by governments are thus excluded from the reach of GATS (for example, Koivusalo, 1999; Pollock and Price, 2000; Hilary, 2001; Lipson, 2001; Sexton, 2001). Koivusalo and Mackintosh (2004: 16) state that "the impact of GATS in health care has so far been limited, though the liberalisation of insurance markets may be increasingly important in health". They further point to the dangers of market failure in the field (for example, exclusion from care owing to inability to pay). More directly connected to the organisation of health care systems is that "the rapidly increasing privatisation of public sector services provision and contractual arrangements in public sector may [...]

change the picture fast creating conditions for increasing the role of private sector actors as well as providing possibilities for competition on government contracting and procurement" (Koivusalo, 1999: 36). Holden (2005: 679) considers that the first steps towards privatisation could already have led to a blurring of public and private boundaries, and thus fall under GATS provisions. Further, there is concern that the health sector itself could be involved in GATS processes, as there have been occasional moves towards that; for example, the US coalition of Service Industries has intended to use GATS negotiations to further US companies' expansion into foreign health care markets (Sexton, 2001; Holden, 2005: 685).

At the same time, a publication by the WHO and WTO (2002: 113) tries to convince us that GATS "leaves countries the flexibility to manage trade in health services in ways that are consistent with national health policy objectives". The fact that certain services are excluded by GATS, namely those "provided in their exercise of government authority", defined as "any service which is supplied neither on a commercial basis nor in competition with one or more service suppliers", does not really provide a safeguard as the critical terms are not defined (WHO and WTO, 2002: 119; Woodward, 2005). It has been argued that for countries that have an internal market in health care, it is not easy to keep that market closed to foreign trade (Lethbridge, 2004: 6).

On TRIPS, the implications for health care centre around issues of patents, copyrights, trademarks and the licensing of pharmaceuticals. It has been argued that TRIPS is an example of an agreement with substantial indirect implications to health and health care systems. The most important of these implications are mediated through pharmaceutical and research policies and technology transfer. TRIPS has further been characterised as not being about liberalisation of services, "but essentially about protection of commercial interests and rights" (Koivusalo and Mackintosh, 2004: 27; see also Lethbridge, 2004, 2005).

In summary, there are indications and arguments for WTO-facilitated trade agreements that have implications for the provision and organisation of health care systems. These have so far been described as being rather speculative; but developments in trade negotiations certainly need to be closely watched in order to prevent detrimental effects. The justification for not considering these issues within the analysis of this book remains, however: the WTO's activities in relation to the health sector are not explicitly policy prescriptions for or production of knowledge about health care systems; rather the connection to health care systems appears indirectly.

3.4   Conclusions: Actors outside the UN as friend or foe

Though not easily comparable, the OECD and WTO both appear as important international organisations where the development of national health care systems is concerned.

The OECD engages explicitly and directly in health care system matters. Since the late 1990s, the OECD has become increasingly important, and has also challenged the WHO's role in speaking about health care systems. While its original activities mainly focused on developing appropriate indicators to deliver health care system related data to its member states, it has extended its qualitative work substantially in describing and providing prescriptions for health care systems. The OECD is less "global" than the UN organisations, and likes to present itself with a careful and neutral position on health care systems (Deacon and Kaasch, 2008; Kaasch, 2010). It makes increasingly important contributions with regard to health care system ideas by explicitly and concretely providing prescriptions to its member states (and to some extent beyond). The OECD has also become an important global health actor, as it has challenged other international organisations (such as the World Bank, the WHO and ILO), and also represents an important partner for collaborations that make global social policy contributions to understanding and (potentially) strengthening health care systems.

The WTO impacts on health care systems more as a side effect of its activities in facilitating more general trade agreements. The WTO is actually not a "health organisation" and never claimed to be. However, its possible application on health policies and its cross-sectoral reach in regulation may have an effect on WTO policies on national health care systems. The case of the WTO shows that indirect prescriptions may evolve as powerfully as direct ones; and that other international organisations' efforts to develop and improve health care systems with a strong emphasis on big risk pools for financing health care provision may be thwarted by WTO trade agreements without that organisation openly and explicitly making a statement about desirable health policies and health care systems.

Nevertheless, while the OECD has systematically expanded its health care system-related activities, and, doing that, has challenged other international organisations' positions in global social policies concerning health care systems; the role of the WTO is much more speculative, but not necessarily less important in effect.

4
The New Centres of Power? G8, G20 and the BRICS and Health Care Systems

4.1 Introduction

In the past few years, it has become evident that, looking for health care system prescriptions at the level of international organisations no longer captures the full picture. It is striking, indeed, that "health care systems" as a matter of international and global concern have found their way onto the agendas of the G8/G20, and the BRICS. In contrast to the more traditional and continuous work of the international organisations (even if characterised by some ups and downs), the attention on health care systems is more prone to quickly changing fashions (and less dependent on permanent contributions and funding that is available through international organisations). At the same time, if an issue such as health care systems takes an important place at a meeting of heads of states or national ministers, the potential for far-reaching and powerful action may be much higher than if attention were coming from the work of international organisations. Particularly interesting is what has been happening at G8 meetings since the 2008 Toyako Summit, when the Japanese government emphasised the importance of health care systems, and had a related report prepared by a group of researchers. This chapter analyses the relative attention that health care systems have received at G8, G20 and BRICS meetings, the changes over time, and the potential for the consideration of health care systems at such meetings to secure a more stable and profound transnational social policy in the field of health care systems more generally.

Before turning to this, however, it needs to be taken into account that, particularly regarding the G8 and G20, an important issue with regard to evaluating their influence and importance in particular policy fields is measured by the extent of commitments made by members of these groups, and the degree to which these commitments are realised and put into effect. This book, however, is primarily about discourses and ideas around health care systems, and to what extent they shape debates and policies at the global health policy level. It is, of course, not irrelevant if, and how, words are put into action and initiatives, but the fact that a country's aid can fall short of prior commitments does not mean anything in terms of an emphasis on or concern about health care systems in more general global health or aid policies.

A complication to be observed with the type of actors addressed in this chapter is, furthermore, that while there are discussions and commitments made at these meetings, the lack of secretariats and common institutions other than summits requires case study or comparative study designs that analyse each of the member states, and/or the processes around each of the summits of such a group. This is, as such, not within the focus of the analysis reported in this book. Also, the sum of what single member states do and say regarding health care systems in a global context does not necessarily add up to "G8 global health policies". The focus here is, instead, on the attention given to health care systems in the history of the processes of different groupings and fora, and this is discussed against the backcloth of multi-actor and multi-sited global health governance regarding health care systems (as it is the case for numerous other health issues). This shall contextualise claims, expectations and criticisms of the involvement of these groups and fora in health care system issues.

4.2   Group of Eight (G8)

Introduction

A short history about the Group of Eight (G8) is as follows. At the time the (then) Group of Six was created in November 1975 in Rambouillet (France), it comprised the United States (US), the United Kingdom (UK), France, Germany, Italy and Japan. The fact that these six countries decided to come together and discuss common challenges happened against the background of the oil shocks of the early 1970s. The countries' intention was to identify common strategies to cope with the crisis. A key social concern at the time was how to deal with high levels of unemployment in crisis-affected economies. In 1976 Canada became part of the group, and in 1998 Russia joined as a member.

The G8 holds a summit each year, where country leaders and representatives discuss common policy issues and make financial commitments to development. Only within the last months, as a consequence of the Ukraine crisis, has the G8 returned to meeting as a Group of Seven (G7) – excluding Russia.

Health at the G8

While the G8 has existed in some form from the mid-1970s onwards, it was only in the mid-1990s that health appeared as an issue at the meetings; and it has not consistently been addressed since then. Initially, the G7/G8 strategy on health was to support existing UN institutions in their work concerning global health issues. This often meant that G8 member states committed extra-budgetary contributions to key organisations that dealt with health issues. However, doubts about the effectiveness of these international organisations (see for example Chapter 2, section 4 on WHO), meant that the G8 also considered alternative ways in which to support global health policies. This is what, amongst other things, generated the idea, and facilitated the establishment of, the Global Fund to Fight AIDS, Malaria and Tuberculosis (see Chapter 5; see also Kirton et al., 2014).

Nevertheless, from the beginning of the 2000s, the G8 has also developed its own initiatives on health (Kirton et al., 2014). Most of the emphasis in the connected plans and initiatives (particularly the G8 African Action Plan (G8, 2002)) focused on particular diseases and health threats. Therefore, such initiatives, both considering the Global Fund (as originally conceived) and G8 members' commitments on health, rather concerned vertical (disease-focused) initiatives than broader health care system needs. Unfortunately, this is even true in the context of the recent outbreak of Ebola – which notably made a number of global actors reconsider the meaning and importance of health care systems in development contexts: the G7 Foreign Ministers' joint Statement on Ebola (G7 Foreign Ministers, 2014, para. 5) merely states that "[w]e express our readiness to assist the affected countries in their fight against Ebola as well as their efforts to cope with Ebola-induced challenges such as shortages in the provision of non-Ebola basic healthcare, shortages in food and budgetary constraints".

Japanese attempts regarding health care systems at G8 level

Nevertheless, even if health care systems were given more prominence at G8 level, it needs to be taken into account that in such a "high-level" political forum, topics and agendas tend to change easily and quickly, for various reasons that are connected to national interests, changing world politics, suddenly emerging problems, risks or threats and so on. For example, while the 2007 G8 Summit in Heiligendamm (Germany) initially focused on health, even health care systems, this was pushed aside by an emerging discourse on environmental issues (following the publication of the Intergovernmental Panel on Climate Change (IPCC)) (IPCC, 2007). The Japanese government, in contrast, was more persistent over the years in its emphasis on health and health care systems. It has favoured and introduced broader concepts of health issues with an emphasis on the importance of appropriate health care systems, and has repeatedly introduced related issues at the G8. The Okinawa meeting in 2000, particularly, included considerable attention to health issues, and acknowledged the link between health and poverty (Kirton et al., 2014).

> Health is a key priority. Good health contributes directly to economic growth whilst poor health drives poverty. Only through sustained action and coherent international co-operation to fully mobilize new and existing medical, technical and financial resources, can we strengthen health delivery systems and reach beyond traditional approaches to break the vicious cycle of disease and poverty.
>
> (G8, para. 26 – quoted in Kirton et al., 2014)

With a particular emphasis on reaching the health MDGs for its next turn of presidency, the Government of Japan, at the Toyako summit, gave special attention to health issues.[1] A meeting of G8 Health Experts (G8 Health Experts, 2008a) was convened on 14–15 February 2008 and Japan gave substantial monetary contributions to the Global Fund. Further commitments to Africa were made at the summit itself. Looking at the content of commitments, particularly with regard to the attention given to health care systems, the 2008 final declaration was focused mainly on vertical initiatives, though.[2] Nevertheless, following the G8 Health Experts Group report *Toyako Framework for Action on Global Health* (G8 Health Experts, 2008b), the declaration, at least, states: "We emphasize the importance of comprehensive approaches to address the strengthening of health care systems including social health protection" (section 46 a).

H8

This development was regarded positively by WHO (WHO, 2008a) and UNICEF (UNICEF, 2008), who also formed part of the so-called H8, a health group also including the World Bank, GAVI, the Global Fund, UNFPA, UNAIDS and the Gates Foundation. The H8's first meeting was held on 19 July 2007, and has been described as an attempt "to harness their combined public-private influence as a counterpoint to the G8" (Brolan et al., 2013). At this meeting there was consensus that strengthening health care systems was important, and "they urged WHO and the World Bank 'to fast-track the completion of the normative framework for health systems strengthening'" (Reich and Takemi, 2009: 511). The initiative of the Japanese could have meant a shift in the global health focus of this important group of countries; and in this emphasis on health care systems, the G8 was also supported by the Task Force on Global Action for Health Strengthening as it released policy recommendations to the G8 for consideration at the 2009 G8 Summit agenda.[3] Despite the sharpening global economic and financial crisis, at that point, health indeed continued to be an important issue at the G8 Meetings,[4] for example the one held in Italy on 8–10 July 2009. A G8 Health Experts' Report *Promoting Global Health*[5] focused on the health MDGs, strengthening health care systems, promoting health as an outcome of all policies, and increasing the quantity and quality of development aid in the field of health. This happened with explicit reference to the World Health Assembly resolutions on primary health care "as a political goal" (sections 13–14) and to social health protection (section 15).

Other G8 countries, though, not necessarily as explicitly in the G8 context as the Japanese government and working group, have also run related initiatives and developed plans. For example, the UK together with Germany and other countries launched an international health partnership,[6] and the UK in 2008 launched a five-year global health strategy (Her Majesty's Government, 2008). In the context of the G8, also, was the Canadian "Muskoka Initiative", with significant commitments on health as part of official development assistance (ODA). However, global health contribution in terms of coordinated action on health care systems remains limited for the G8. That the focus at the time of writing is once again on other issues than health caused by the Ukraine crisis, and the resulting tensions between the G7 and Russia. The planned 2014 Sochi summit was cancelled, and instead a G7 meeting was held in Brussels in June 2014, but global health was not particularly high on the agenda. In terms of the focus on health this is a depressing development, as some experts had expectations regarding the Sochi summit, because of the earlier interest of Russia in the G8 on health issues. In February 2014, the first G8 Health Experts' Group (HEG) meeting was indeed held in Moscow.[7] However, the focus would not have been on health care systems, most certainly, but on the fight against infectious diseases, the availability of vaccines and treatment, lack of essential health care services, and the shortage and migration of health care workers (see Kulik, 2011: 4). A continued dramatic spread of Ebola, though, might threaten G8 countries enough to focus on necessary health measures, and possibly this would bring health care systems back to the G8 agenda.

The G8's transformative power

In general it can be said that the political power, the visibility and flexibility that the G8 (Reich and Takemi, 2009: 512) provides as a forum and changer in issues related to health care systems is diminished because health care systems easily slip down the agenda once another crisis seems to be more important – either another policy field (environmental issues), or a global economic crisis that – particularly regarding the one that started in 2008 – leads to silence on health care systems rather than a changed global discourse that puts health care systems in the centre of a general debate about austerity. This was expressed by Japan's prime minister, Shinzo Abe, who wrote in the *Lancet*:

> At the G8 Hokkaido Toyako Summit in 2008, Japan proposed a comprehensive approach to health, inclusive of health system strengthening, to complement a vertical approach. [...] Unfortunately, because of the financial crisis [...], there have

been difficulties in sustaining the amount of aid for health. We should now pursue universal health coverage (UHC) to solve existing global health challenges and to embark on the post-2015 development agenda.

(Abe, 2013: 915)

It is worth, though, taking a closer look at the policy papers prepared by the Takemi Working Group as something that could, if taken up again, usefully guide the G8's engagement in health care systems as part of its broader global health and development initiatives (for an overview and discussion see Reich and Takemi, 2009). This is of course also true regarding the G8's involvement in the process of developing future development goals.

On a positive note the G8 process "provides a highly personal, visible and flexible mechanism for addressing global health policy making" (Reich and Takemi, 2009: 512) – apart from obvious issues of implementation capacity and the dependence on other organisations and institutions for concretising and realising concepts, ideas and plans: the development of such plans and ideas is subject to high fluidity and is therefore not very coherent or reliable. The question, as asked by Chand et al. (2010: 1), remains: "does a consensus exist in the G8 to take on the nuanced issues of health systems strengthening, or to get the G20 involved?"

4.3   Between G8 and G20: The BRICS as the new global health actor?

Before turning to the role of the G20, it is useful to consider the meaning of the BRICS group of countries in order to capture the increasingly important role of the "countries of the South". BRICS stands for Brazil, Russia, India, China and South Africa. In 2006, the first four countries began to meet as a group; in 2011 South Africa joined. It is obvious what brings these countries together: they are all increasingly powerful global economies, and they form their political and economic interest to some extent in competition with the traditionally strong economies of Western Europe and North America.

[. . .] BRICS represent a block of countries with a [. . .] great potential to move global public health in the right

direction... towards reducing the current vast gaps in health outcomes and introducing greater fairness in the way the benefits of
medical and scientific progress are distributed [...]

(Chan, 2011: para. 53)

Less obvious is what defines their joint activities or advocacy, in
health policy as in other fields. The countries' activities are in the first
place, probably even more than the G8, driven by individual domestic conditions and interests, more than truly common ideas about, or
even an interest in, how to make the world a more social place. Furthermore, the activities themselves, so far, happen primarily on an
ad-hoc basis, but one can also observe continuous efforts to develop
more formal mechanisms for collaboration.

It needs to be taken into account, in trying to understand the
role of BRICS as a global health actor, that these countries continue to appear to be emerging economies that still have quite some
way to go in order to make their own health care systems work
well and respond to problems of poverty, inequality and the related
health needs of their populations. At the same time these countries
increasingly act as donors and foreign shapers of other countries'
national policies within contexts of global governance. While the
BRICS countries' contribution to foreign assistance is, so far, comparatively small, it is significantly increasing. Nevertheless "their interest
and goals in supporting global health and development efforts are
tempered by domestic concerns" (Global Health Strategies Initiative,
2012: 6). Civil society organisations also alert us to the fact that the
way the BRICS approach foreign aid is different from the approaches
of "traditional" donors: based on a self-perception of already having made significant achievements in the field of health, the BRICS
regard themselves as particularly suitable to "teach" other developing
countries how to approach particular health policies. Even more, they
consider cooperation and mutual support on a "South-South" basis
particularly promising and justified. The different BRICS countries
each follow their own specific ideas and approaches in development
aid, but common to all of them is an emphasis on bilateral capacity building and infrastructure development (Global Health Strategies
Initiative, 2012).

On health more specifically, the contributions of BRICS include
knowledge production and advocacy, and addressing social and

health policy issues in meetings, declarations and action plans (see Surender and Urbina-Ferretjans, 2015). Apart from international political gatherings, knowledge production and the development of joint visions also happens in the so-called "BRICS Academic Forums". Harmer et al. (2013) distinguish ideational, institutional and material influence, as well as the different modes, sources and reasons for BRICS influence on global health in reviewing the literature.

Historically, there were first health commitments by the BRICS at a South Africa meeting in 2011, which focused on the dialogue and cooperation in social protection, and doing this included public health and particularly measures against HIV/AIDS. This was accompanied by a commitment to a first meeting of health ministers, which happened some months later. At that meeting the importance of (strengthening) health care systems was acknowledged, and further meetings were planned. Since 2011, BRICS health ministers have been meeting, sidelining the WHO's World Health Assemblies.

Emerging from the first meetings on health, the so-called "Beijing Declaration" made a number of important points concerning health systems.[8] section 6 of the declaration says:

> The strengthening of health systems and health financing in developing countries in all regions must be the central goal of the global health community. In our view, WHO has a major role to play in the promotion of access to medication, technology transfer and capacity-building with a view to bring more equity to the health sector worldwide. Success in health outcomes in our country represents success to many others.

Among the priority areas for collaborative action agreed upon, the BRICS highlight strengthening health systems and increasing access to "medical products", and collaboration with a number of other global health actors (section 10).

Therefore, it has become evident that the BRICS, indeed, go beyond single member states' activities, and have begun acting as a group in the field of health. However, in 2012, CSOs commented that the "BRICS have declared health collaboration a priority, but they have not yet begun to work collectively to enhance the impact of their assistance programs" (Global Health Strategies Initiative, 2012). Meanwhile, at the 2013 meeting, the "BRICS Framework on

Collaboration on Strategic Projects in Health" was adopted.[9] In this "Joint Communiqué of the BRICS Member States on Health on the Sidelines of the 67th World Health Assembly", "universal health coverage" is mentioned as a key thematic focus area on which to collaborate, as well as reference being made to the health-related MDGs. It is "emphasized that discussions on Universal Health Coverage must encompass strengthening national health systems and addressing human resources for health, which are essential for the fulfilment of the right to health and wellbeing for all" (section 4).

The real impact of such health statements and the BRICS impact on the global health landscape and national health policies in their own and other developing countries will still have to be seen. The BRICS leaders seem to be convinced about the BRICS' position: according to a joint explanation of BRICS health collaboration, the "BRICS are truly contributing to reshaping the international health-cooperation landscape" (Barbosa da Silva et al., 2014: 388). While the five thematic areas mentioned here do not seem to include health care systems as such (only the strengthening of health surveillance systems is mentioned), the three tracks of work for collaboration that emerged from the meeting in Cape Town, South Africa, in November 2013 include health care systems – again with an emphasis on "the importance of monitoring and evaluating progress towards universal health coverage" (Barbosa da Silva et al., 2014: 388). The paper concludes:

> In short, much depends on these elements to elucidate universal health coverage of preventive, diagnostic, therapeutic, rehabilitative and caring services for the increasing burden of co-morbidities due to communicable and non-communicable diseases, as well as accidents, will be a global reality.
>
> (Barbosa da Silva et al., 2014: 388)

Accordingly, the BRICS are developing a Monitoring and Evaluation Tool for Universal Health Coverage.

Furthermore, even if the development of a guiding concept might not have emerged so far, other global health actors such as the WHO and UNAIDS have explicitly acknowledged the BRICS group as a new global health actor (see also Surender and Urbina-Ferretjans, 2015). The BRICS also interact with the Global Fund (see Chapter 5).

4.4   Group of Twenty (G20)

The G20 is comprised of the G8 members (Canada, France, Germany, Italy, Japan, Russia, the UK and the US), the BRICS members (Brazil, [Russia], India, China and South Africa) and Argentina, Australia, Indonesia, Mexico, the Republic of Korea, Saudi Arabia, Turkey and the European Union (EU). In that it includes more of the world's developed and emerging economies, it has become increasingly the focus of a promising step towards more inclusive modes of global governance. Furthermore, it has shown to be a place for social policy issues since the G20 became ever more important in the context of the global economic and financial crisis, from about 2008 onwards.

It was in 1999 that the G20 finance ministers gathered for the first time to discuss issues of market access, investment and economic stability. Since the G20 became more important and powerful, particularly following the beginning of the global economic and financial crisis, there has been a discussion about the G20 replacing the G8. Particularly given the current struggles around the role of Russia in the Ukraine conflict, such issues are currently in the background of public and political debate. In terms of economic power, though, the relevance of the G7/G8 as a leading group of countries has been increasingly questioned (debates about the representation of emerging economies in the international financial institutions being another expression of this).

As for the other groups of countries, there is no permanent secretariat but it is the respective summit host's responsibility to set agendas and organise the meetings. As such, the G20 is a network with the aim of gaining consensus on a number of shared policy concerns and issues. In publicly announcing these, it may have political authority. It is hard, however, to clearly figure out concrete interests and mandates over a longer period (Chand et al., 2010: 2).

Regarding health policies, the G20 has not yet gone beyond recognising public health in "the importance of strengthening social safety nets like public health care" (Kulik, 2011: 5). Not even in the interesting governance structure sidelining the G20 general summits, namely, the L20,[10] Y20[11] and C20[12] summits, we can identify a major interest in, or push for, including health policies or health care systems. At a conference at Chatham House,[13] it was suggested that the difference partly stems from the fact that G8 sherpas know each other personally and had a joint incentive to work out a meaningful communiqué for health. A similar approach is much more difficult in a G20 context, even if only because of the larger number of delegates.

4.5 Conclusions: Varying importance of global groups and forums

It is important to acknowledge that, as opposed to an international organisation or the Global Fund (to be addressed in the following chapter), the groups of countries discussed in this chapter use their meetings as opportunities to discuss strategies and sometimes to make commitments, but in the end they still act more as states than as a group. This does not make them less powerful, though. It does, however, have implications for the attention and meaning given to a topic such as health care systems, if such groups appear as increasingly important actors in global social and health governance. The implications can be different, both positive and negative for the global governance of health care systems, and at different levels of health policymaking.

There have been discussions about these actors' responsibility for addressing health care systems, as, institutionally, it is obvious they are not able to fulfil any meaningful, sustainable and coherent role in supporting health care systems. This is because these groups of countries do not have secretariats, but are structured by changing hosts (rotating chairs) who also define the agenda. Health care systems may be a topic and have been a topic at some times (during health crises), or may be in the particular interest of one or a few countries (such as Japan), but the prominence of other topics (such as climate change) or other crises (for example, the global economic and financial crisis of 2008 onwards) may also mean that even health policies more broadly (not only health care systems) are completely off the agenda.

Nevertheless, we see a major difference in the attention given to health care systems between the smaller G8 and BRICS, which have engaged explicitly and increasingly with health care systems, and the G20 – to some extent combining and extending the two groups – which has not meaningfully addressed the issue. Also, Kirton et al. have remarked the contrast between the BRICS engagement in health and that at both G8 and G20 levels (Kirton et al., 2014).

While not having been systematically included in the study reported here, it should be mentioned that the World Economic Forum (WEF) and the World Social Forum (WSF) are also potential and actual fora for discussing health care systems among global actors. For example, the WEF features a "Health for All" strategy, including the issue of health care delivery models, and the discussion at the WEF 2009 stressed the importance of questions about the delivery of health care (presented as a shift in focus from insurance questions).[14] Being primarily a platform of discussion without political decisions taken, the health care system position at such meetings may have an impact on actors that otherwise would not consider health care systems to be an issue.

Parallel to the WEF, the WSF as a gathering of civil society organisations has been a venue for many advocacy activities to make a start, also with regard to health care systems. For example, the WSF in 2007 included discussions about the human right to health and the creation and development of universal, comprehensive and equitable health care systems and social security in the African and world context.[15]

5
The Global Fund to Fight AIDS, Tuberculosis and Malaria: A Hybrid Organisation as the Best Health Care System Actor?

5.1 Introduction

Another global health actor that has been faced with considerable and varying expectations of its role and importance in speaking on and for health care systems has been, since the early 2000s, the Global Fund to Fight AIDS, Tuberculosis and Malaria (Global Fund). Born out of a number of developments, and originally focused on three particular communicable diseases (thus driven by a "vertical" logic), over the years, the Global Fund has also assumed a role regarding health care systems.

This chapter investigates to what extent the Global Fund has been expected to take on, and has taken on, a role in health care systems, adding to its attempts to fight three specific diseases. It also considers to what extent the global economic and financial crisis from 2008 onwards has changed the importance of the Global Fund, and in particular, how this has affected the focus on health care systems in Global Fund activities.

In the previous chapter, it was indicated that part of the "health contribution" that stemmed from the G8 was support of the Global Fund. This was created in 2002 as an outcome of a Special Session on HIV/AIDS by the UN General Assembly. However, other global institutions and events also played a role, such as meeting the targets of the MDGs, the Abuja Declaration, the Report of the Commission on Macroeconomics and Health (see also Chapter 2, section 4) and the G8 meeting in Okinawa that eventually came up with the idea of a new financing mechanism (Bartsch, 2005).

The Global Fund was originally designed as a *pure* financing mechanism to increase and manage development aid to the health sector, directed to a small number of diseases. It has, however, developed into a global social policy actor relevant for health care systems. The Global Fund deliberately focused on three major global diseases, as the idea was to use it to attract and disburse additional resources for fighting these diseases (Hanefeld, 2011: 161). It was set up as a "public-private partnership" – with the intention of establishing a new "mechanism" (rather than a new "organisation"), involving governments, civil society, the private sector and affected communities. This public-private partnership comprises governments, civil society, the private sector and affected communities. It was conceived not as a new form of "international organisation" but as a "new approach to international health financing" or a "funding mechanism" (not an implementing agency).[1] However, at the same time, and in contrast to the groups of countries described above, it has a secretariat to inform, guide and realise its activities. The Global Fund's main purpose, at its foundation, was to attract and disburse (additional) resources to fight HIV/AIDS, tuberculosis and malaria.

The Global Fund is administered by a limited number of staff. Administration was initially integrated into the WHO, but later it was run independently, and the Global Fund now operates from a secretariat in Geneva. The Global Fund's Executive Board is responsible for developing strategies, policies, operational guidelines and funding decisions. Groups represented are the donors (eight representatives of industrialised countries and two representatives of the private sector) and the recipients (seven representatives of developing countries and three civil society representatives) as voting members. Non-voting members are three representatives of international organisations (WHO, UNAIDS, World Bank) and a Swiss member (Bartsch, 2005).

The Executive Board reviews grant applications, and grants are awarded on a competitive basis directly to countries. This also means that there are no national representations of the Global Fund in countries. The grants are given to so-called principal recipients, including government ministries, NGOs and research institutions (Hanefeld, 2011: 162). The grant applications are developed through a Country Coordination Mechanism (CCM) including the representation of all sections of society. That implies that the "CCM prepares the proposals based on local needs and gaps in national programmes" (Dräger et al., 2006). This is then evaluated by the Global Fund's Technical Review Panel (appointed by the Global Fund's Board, and comprising international health and development experts).

5.2 The Global Fund and health care systems

This structure is intended to facilitate two key principles: that of country ownership and that of performance-based funding. In their original sense, these principles rather contradicted any function of health care system prescriptions. The focus on three diseases also supported a "vertical approach" logic. Nevertheless, after some years of Global Fund activity, and just before the global economic and financial crisis struck, claims to broaden its mandate were raised.

Dräger et al. (2006) reported a study of the Global Fund's long-term effects on health care systems, undertaken by the "Systemwide Effects of the Fund (SWEF) Research Network". They reviewed the evolving health care system engagement of the Global Fund by studying the guidance notes for grant seeking provided by the Global Fund secretariat. According to their findings, there was considerable concern in the first round about the "institutional and absorptive capacity" in a country; later on, increasingly the emphasis was on an integrated approach with regard to health care systems and vertical, disease-related measures (Dräger et al., 2006).

A team of experts warned that there was a risk of "Medicines without Doctors" if the Fund did not take into account health sector scale up (Ooms et al., 2007). Furthermore, these experts claimed that the Global Fund (not the World Bank) would be best placed to strengthen health care systems. Indeed, in November 2007, the Board of the Global Fund approved US$1 billion in new grants, out of which nearly 20 per cent would be contributed to large-scale strengthening of in-country health care systems. When the Global Fund was evaluated in 2009, it was concluded that it was a "major investor in health systems" and had also indirectly strengthened health care systems through its activities.[2]

Looking at the Strategic Objectives in the new strategy for 2012–2016, we find plans to "maximize the impact of the Global Fund investment on strengthening health systems [and] on improving the health of mothers and children", to "integrate human rights consid-erations [...], [and] increase investments in programs that address human rights-related barriers to access" (The Global Fund, 2012). This suggests that health care systems continue to be an issue for the Global Fund.

However, the Global Fund has also struggled with the implications of the global financial crisis which limited its scope of activities, mak-ing it more likely that the Global Fund will have to diminish the role of broader health care system support in its activities. Furthermore, it had some of its contributions suspended in 2012 owing to issues of corruption that had to be investigated.

After the meeting in November 2012 and the approval of US$1 billion in new grants, (out of which nearly 20 per cent were supposed to contribute to large-scale strengthening of in-country health care systems through upgrading infrastructure, strengthening essential procurement and supply management systems, reinforcing human resources and buying new health equipment), at the fourth replen-ishment in December 2013, "the largest amount ever committed to fight against AIDS, tuberculosis and malaria" was pledged.[3]

In terms of the concrete development of an appropriate way of engaging with health care systems, and taking to heart the earlier expert advice concerning more emphasis on health care systems, the Global Fund asked the WHO for advice on the issue. This led to a report entitled "The Global Fund Strategic Approach to Health Sys-tems Strengthening" (WHO, 2007b). The WHO's recommendations include the use of an "HSS floor",[4] "possibly as a percentage of any grant, [that] might be more useful to help promote the desired 'diag-onal' approach".[5] While the approach of an HSS fund can be found to be part of the Global Fund's declared activities, it is interesting to see that there are now, in the context of the Ebola crisis, voices that are calling for a new fund, rather than a reload of the Global Fund's responsibility for health care systems.

5.3   Conclusions

This development of the Global Fund during about one and a half decades suggests that a concern about health care systems has indeed taken hold in the functioning of the organisation. Thereby, WHO advice (between global actors) has had an important impact on the ideas of health care systems included in Global Fund activities. A separate study would have to explore the extent to which that is successful, and if it means a promising change in the way global health projects and health-related development aid are approached.

6
Non-Governmental Organisations and Health Care System Ideas

6.1 Introduction

The picture of global social policy in the field of health care systems is even more complex when taking into account yet other global health actors, such as business organisations and civil society organisations (CSOs). Given the specific focus of this book, namely on models of health care systems, the number of such non-governmental actors, generating and disseminating knowledge and ideas on health care systems, and being able to join in related discourses, is much smaller, though. On the one hand, among business actors, for example, health receives relatively little attention (Farnsworth, 2005: 75); and business actors impact on health care systems instead through other related policy fields, rather than through a direct engagement in the health sector (via insurance companies, pharmaceutical companies and so on). These actors might, however, also have an impact on supranational health regulations, and may try to influence trade agreements in their own interest. Looking at CSOs, many of their activities are either concentrated on very specific health issues, in specific regions, or such organisations may be primarily active in on-the-ground activities (for example in the direct provision of health services and medicines). CSOs might be directly engaged with international organisations, and might try to influence their ideas and activities. However, their scope for producing comprehensive or complex ideas, models and reform suggestions for health care systems independently appears to be rather limited.

This chapter nevertheless engages with the role of CSOs by focusing on one particularly interesting initiative, namely the production and content of the so-called Global Health Watch, compiled by a group of non-governmental organisations as a sort of "alternative world health report". The chapter first briefly discusses the role of CSOs in global social and health policy in general and then illustrates such activities with a detailed analysis and discussion of the Global Health Watch initiative and the models proposed in their reports. Doing that, it needs to be taken into account that the focus of this chapter is on the roles of CSOs as *compared to* and *in relation to* international organisations, even more complex systems of multi-actored global social governance; not – as for example in Lee's contribution (2007) – the role of CSOs *in* international organisations.

6.2 Civil society organisations as global social policy actors

CSOs are often understood as the "third system" of global actors (besides international organisations and business actors). Following Florini (2000b), the term CSO refers to self-organised advocacy groups, undertaking collective action in pursuit of a defined public interest (see also Price, 2003). Such collective action may include the development and dissemination of ideas, projects, campaigns and so on.

"Transnational civil society networks are often quite effective at portraying themselves as doers of the good" (Florini, 2000a: 231), and equally, the literature on CSOs is often predominantly positive about their contributions to global governance (for example, Williams and Young, 1994). However, using terms from peace and conflict studies, CSOs can be "a factor in war as well as a force for peace" (Barnes, 2005). They are identified as contributing to more democratic development; providing development alternatives (Drabek, 1987; Clark, 1991; Farrington and Bebbington, 1993); mobilising, articulating and representing people's interests at different levels of decision-making (Jordan and van Tuijl, 2000: 2051); and representing agents of accountability (Fox and Brown, 1998). At the same time, critical aspects of the role of CSOs have also been pointed to, regarding, amongst other things, their performance, accountability and transparency (for example, Jordan and van Tuijl, 2000; Bebbington, 2004, 2005). Yet others have seen potential damage through CSOs, as they can "inadvertently contribute to exacerbate division and tensions among actors by inadequate analysis and inadequate skills, or becoming advocates for one side" ("Do no harm" programme of the Collaborative for Development Action),[1] or a "wrong" side (Florini, 2000a). Teegen et al. (2004: 471) also mention that CSOs "may compromise their effectiveness if they [...] tackle issues that are too complex".[2]

The attention given to NGOs or CSOs by global social policy literature is not impressive, as has been brought forward as an issue by Yeates (2001). A chapter by Kruse and Martens (2015) goes some steps further in the matter, but they do not provide for a case study that applies some of the points made about the roles of this type of actor in global social policy prescriptions.

If CSOs are able to fulfil a role in providing alternative models of health care systems, their mandates and legitimacy to do that, are – for most of them – not comparable with those of the international (governmental) organisations discussed above. Nevertheless, CSOs fulfil functions of research and development (R&D); advocacy; as "proponents" as well as "protagonists" of specific ideas (Delisle, et al. 2005; Abbott, 2007; Bartsch, 2007). While several CSOs are said to have had impressive records in global health research, there are differences in research approaches in comparison to more academic work that is a part of the publications emanating from international organisations. There are also particular constraints on this type of actor in justifying extensive research activity as the funding they have, often donations, is usually given for more direct health or aid intervention (Delisle et al., 2005).

6.3   The Global Health Watch: A viable alternative for health care systems?

Organisation

The initiative of the Global Health Watch is an exception among CSOs in that it develops such a comprehensive concept of health care systems and provides for complex recommendations on the matter. Up to now, the initiative has comprised a number of NGOs, and has produced three Global Health Watches that are supposed to represent and function as "alternative world health reports".[3] Therefore, the Global Health Watch initiative serves as the case study for this analysis of the role of CSOs in the global discourse on health care systems.

The Global Health Watch is an initiative and the product of a civil society movement in health. It operates as a platform for CSOs and individuals working in health and health-related sectors. As a report, it is compiled as a collaboration of several CSOs, including the People's Health Movement (PHM), Medact, the Global Equity Gauge (GEGA), the Third World Network, Health Action International and Centre de Estudios y Asesoria en Salud (CEAS). Its coordinating committee consists of academics, health activists and public health practitioners from different regions of the world. The first report was published in 2005, the second in 2008 and the third in 2011. For the production of these reports, the secretariat has moved from the UK to South Africa to India.[4]

Global Health Watch is a mobilisation and advocacy instrument in that it is supposed to be "a call for action written in a clear, accessible style to appeal to grass-roots health workers and activists worldwide, as well as to international policy-makers and national decision makers" (Global Health Watch, 2005: i). While at first glance this appears to be a rather broad range of possible recipients, the professional groups that are given as examples (health workers, teachers, engineers, geographers, farmers and biologists) to fulfil the universal right to health and dignity (Global Health Watch, 2005: 4), suggests an organisation along epistemic community lines (Haas, 1992). Other professional groups such as health economists or lawyers are not mentioned, even though they might also be engaged in furthering human development and social justice.

The different organisations and individuals working together on this project share a basic view about the current situation of global health governance. The common general mission and aims include the promotion of human rights as a basis for health policy; to provide an alternative to liberal and market-driven perspectives; and to claim increased recognition of the political, social and economic barriers to better health in health policy agendas.[5] The concern goes beyond specific health needs towards a view on inequalities (see Global Health Watch 2, 2009: 2).

The organisations and individuals that have gathered to compile the Global Health Watch can be usefully understood through the concept of transnational advocacy networks or coalitions (Keck and

Sikkink, 1998; Stone, 2002). The participants (organisations and individuals) are "bound together by shared values, [...] and a shared discourse" (Stone, 2002: 4), while not dependent on "the status of recognized professional status of 'experts' " (Stone, 2002: 4). Their binding element is "principled beliefs" in the sense of "normative ideas that provide criteria to distinguish right from wrong". For the Global Health Watch those joint principled beliefs concern a particular definition of the Alma-Ata principles; while these in fact have always been subject to different interpretations by different actors and at different times. The intention of the initiative is, in theoretical terms, to "shape the climate of public debate and influence global policy agendas" (Stone, 2002: 4). This is done by providing for specific interpretations, explanations and suggestions about a range of global health topics, including health care systems, and actors (international organisations impacting on health policy). Doing this, CSOs, among them the Global Health Watch initiative, "are mechanisms with which to broadcast and advocate one form of knowledge, [...] or norms in preference of other perspectives" (Stone, 2002: 6). Kaldor describes such groups as "a new form of global politics that parallels and supplements formal democracy at the national level" (2003: 107).

However, being concerned with a particular policy field and dimension of global health governance, it is also important to take into consideration the content of their ideas or advice (Deacon et al., 1997). The pure fact that advocacy coalitions fulfil specific roles, or in the case of the Global Health Watch pursue a certain set of health objectives, does not yet tell us anything about the extent to which this is justified. To examine this, it is essential to observe *what* these groups are saying and claiming, in combination with their potential or actual power to disseminate such ideas and their likely influence in changing the ideas of others.

The Global Health Watches ideas on health care systems

The Global Health Watch provides for both the presentation and discussion of a number of global health policy topics, and the articulation of alternative models and views on those topics, as well as the surveillance of activities of the major international organisations engaged in health. The report is understood as an "alternative world health report" written with the aim of providing "hard-hitting, evidence-based analysis of the political economy of health and health care – as a challenge to the major global bodies that influence health" (Global Health Watch, 2005: i). It includes concrete actions for everybody, as well as recommendations for a better global health governance.

The three editions of the Global Health Watch address a number of global health topics and functions, while in this book the focus is on ideas about health care systems only. The reports' basic underlying approach is an understanding of health that is explicitly political and also comprehensive (including poverty), as well as being interested in equity and rights, in a broad sense, including (besides political and civil liberty human rights) social, economic and cultural rights.

Health care systems are addressed explicitly and comprehensively, including their different functions. Based on the observation that there are still millions of people without access to health care because of non-existent, weak or struggling health care systems, the three reports develop an agenda for health care system development going back to the Alma-Ata Declaration (WHO/UNICEF, 1978). The Declaration's principles are presented and interpreted as follows: a comprehensive approach to health, emphasising preventive interventions and promoting a multisectoral approach; the integration of different clinical services and different levels of health care; an emphasis on equity; the use of "appropriate" health technology (socially and culturally acceptable); appropriate community involvement; and a strong human rights perspective.

At the same time, similar to the hesitation to prescribe one-size-fits-all models imposed by international organisations, we can read in the second Global Health Watch:

> There are no quick-fix solutions: Strengthening health systems requires a multidimensional programme of change and development, guided by a long-term vision. It also requires a set of guiding principles, specifically around:
>
> - progressive health financing;
> - pooling health finance to optimize risk-sharing and cross-subsidisation;
> - fitting health-care expenditure and utilization patterns according to need, rather than demand or the ability to pay;

- balancing population-based approaches to health with individualized health care;
- balancing needs-driven and rights-based health provision against commercialization.

(Global Health Watch 2, 2009: 38)

However, the District Health System (DHS) model, developed by the WHO following the Alma-Ata conference, is described in the Global Health Watch reports as a model to realise these principles within the health care system. The DHS is characterised by clearly demarcated geographical areas. It provides the basis for the integration of different level health services; it is coordinated with other key sectors (for example, water); and is organised by a district-level management team concerned about comprehensive and integrated health care. The report continues to provide a number of far-reaching recommendations to "restore a proper balance and relationship between the public and private sectors as well as between public health care (population and community-based approaches to health) and individual private health care" (Global Health Watch, 2005: 79). The public sector is said to have the central role in this process. Ten recommendations are developed that need to be implemented together, and adjusted to the particular context in a given country. Specifically, on the main functions of health care systems (financing, provision, regulation), it is stated that there is a general stress on the role of the public sector in all three functions. Regarding financing, a single national pool is the aim, "with the capacity for cross-subsidization between high-income and low-income groups, and risk sharing between, for example, the young and the elderly" (Global Health Watch, 2005). For low-income countries, there is further a dimension of external financing that must happen through debt relief and medium- and long-term external financing, channelled through Ministries of Health. If there are private providers, the choice should be on non-profit providers. Strong and clear national regulation is necessary, with community involvement. The DHS is presented as the model to fulfil these functions, as:

> It creates a decentralized system to allow health plans and programmes to be tailored to the needs and characteristics of the local population and topography. It provides a platform for the

integration of policies and priorities emanating from different programmes and initiatives at the central level, and for getting the appropriate balance between top-down and bottom-up planning. Districts can form the basis for resource-allocation decisions informed by a population-based assessment of need, and can help central levels of the health care system to identify areas requiring additional capacity development or support.

(Global Health Watch, 2005: 92)

Compared to the models promoted by international organisations which have been discussed in chapters 2 and 3, the Global Health Watch's DHS model is much more focused on provision and explicitly favours a decentralised approach to provision, as well as participation in decision-making (Global Health Watch, 2005). Furthermore, Global Health Watch 2 explains:

Ideally, service providers would be adequately paid through a system that delinks their income from the delivery of health care (a critical condition for ethical behavior and values within health care systems), whilst encouraging quality and responsiveness through monitoring and evaluation, competition for non-financial rewards, fostering a culture of excellence and community empowerment.

(Global Health Watch 2, 2009: 38)

The approach suggested in the Global Health Watches shows a strong emphasis on the public sector and supports one single public pool for health care financing (Global Health Watch, 2004: 5). However, the financing model claimed for goes far beyond the national level:

An adequate human infrastructure for health systems in low-income countries will require increased levels of health expenditure. There are three possible strategies. First, low-income countries can improve health expenditure by increasing their public budgets through more efficient and effective systems, and then allocating a higher proportion of the public budget to health. Second, high-income countries could reach the long-standing target of allocating 0.7 per cent of gross national income (GNI) to development assistance, and commit to reliable transfer of funds for periods of five to ten years. Third, in a globalized world economy, public finance should be generated at the global level, possibly through an international tax authority of some sort that could help reclaim the hundreds of billions of dollars of public revenue lost due to tax avoidance and tax competition (Tax Justice Network, 2007).[6] In addition to generating revenue for health and poverty eradication, regulation of global finance and banking could help reduce levels of corruption.

(Global Health Watch 2, 2009: 40; footnote added)

The following Global Health Watch 3 is perhaps a bit less convinced of the chance to bring together these different levels of solidarity and redistribution. It still stresses "*a* need to press for more international aid", but also states that "funding at the domestic level must be harnessed" (Global Health Watch 3, 2011: 63). Regarding the generation of financing universal coverage at the domestic level, Global Health Watch 3 engages with best financing mechanisms and how to address equity and universal coverage. Unsurprisingly, user fees are rejected. Insurance systems are not as clearly rejected, but "the clear prescription is towards a public, fax-financed system" (particularly Global Health Watch 3, 2011: 71ff.).

While some of the elements of the model prescribed come close to those favoured by the major health international organisations, the WHO and the World Bank, particularly the idea of one pool for financing health care, what the Global Health Watches call for differs remarkably. They stress the role of the public and non-profit sector in health care provision, as well as the importance of community involvement in regulation. Interestingly, national governments are not the only units to be suggested as responsible for realising a sustainable health care system: "Governments, multinational corporations and citizens have duties and obligations to people within and across national boundaries to achieve the universal attainment of human rights" (Global Health Watch 2, 2009: 2).

Concerning the health work of other global health actors – and given that the aim is also to "watch" the other global health actors, particularly the major international organisations – the reports tend to be driven by a historical perspective, with preconceived conceptions about the different international organisations engaged in, or impacting on, health care systems. This tends to result in the WHO being given the central and most justified role, while dismissing the World Bank. For example, Global Health Watch 1 tells the story of the detrimental effects of the World Bank's and the IMF's structural adjustment programmes and conditional loans on national health care systems. The World Bank is further associated with the promotion of user fees, and as a proponent of private systems for all but the poor, referring to the IFC's activities and a paper by Gwatkin.[7]

The more problematic side of the information provided in the publication concerns the picture drawn of some of the other global health actors, for example the World Bank and its – alleged – ideas and role in the guidance of national health care systems. The information given in this case is at best extremely one-sided. As has been demonstrated in the contribution by Shaw (2007), the World Bank has learned from mistakes made in the past; and it is extremely complex as an organisation as well as in its output of policy ideas. While the work cited in the Global Health Watch is certainly one side of the World Bank (Group), it does not do justice to the complexity of the organisation and the quality of health research that is also undertaken by the World Bank (some of which has been described in Chapter 2 of this book). Assuming the potential power of CSOs in shaping global health discourse and in global health governance, the accuracy and quality of the information provided *does* matter. This is not to say that there should not be space for variation and dissent regarding the assessment of global health problems, the interpretation of specific interventions or opinions about desirable health care systems. However, mobilisation on the ground of one-sided or even wrong information could be dangerous; and well-intended pressure by CSOs does not always produce the right outcome, as has also been shown in Shaw's (2007) contribution.

6.4   Conclusions: The Global Health Watch as an important alternative or one-sided element of resistance?

From the above descriptions, the Global Health Watch appears indeed to be a CSO instrument that provides for alternative policy ideas at the global health level; and provides for an alternative health care system model. Concerning the characterisation of other global health actors, it is driven by preconceived opinions, rather than carefully studying particular health topics.

A critical note concerns the lack of sufficient evidence for some of the statements made – even if this is understandable to some extent. Sections such as the following paint the report in a light that is not much better than those that the Global Health Watches criticise:

> There is compelling **anecdotal** evidence that these target-driven, performance-based funding mechanisms pressurize countries to "focus on more easily reached target populations and politically high profile treatment campaigns, thereby exacerbating inequalities, neglecting population-wide public health programmes" (Brugha, 2008),[8] including shifting health personnel away from general health care, and fragmenting services into a set of parallel "vertical" programmes.
>
> (Global Health Watch 3, 2011: 48, emphasis and footnote added)

The Global Health Watch as a project, a group of CSOs, as well as a document is certainly an example of both the good and the problematic sides of CSOs' engagement in global health governance. In terms of the policy model presented, indeed, it provides for an alternative concept of desirable health care systems, in a global health topic that is otherwise characterised by similar models (Kaasch, 2007). The ideas presented in the Global Health Watch prioritise important social goals and the role of the public sector in health governance much more strongly than is the case in the concepts provided by the major international organisations in the field. In bringing together groups and individuals sharing the same set of values, it further provides a mechanism of strengthening the voice of progressive CSOs within global health discourse. In this sense, the Global Health Watch is an important contribution to global health governance in guiding national health care systems.

7
The Polish Health Care System Under Global Scrutiny

7.1 Introduction

So far, this book has focused on actors, ideas and exchanges at global – or transnational – policy levels only. Making direct connections between global discursive spheres and national social or health policy reforms is a difficult task. It has, however, been shown in numerous studies that particular groups of countries, at particular historical times, have been prone to significant external influence in their social and health policies. These have taken different shapes, including contextual influences, policy learning and conditional aid. The organisations and their ideas and activities discussed above relate to national health care systems, on the one hand, through possible application of the general concepts (undertaken by national policymakers and bureaucrats); but on the other hand, the organisations also apply their work to specific countries in separate publications, programmes, country loans and so on.

One group of countries that has been particularly focused on by international organisations and other actors are the formerly Communist Central and Eastern European countries, also referred to as transition countries. Particularly in times of crisis and while general restructuring of political systems and institutions is going on, it is common for national policymakers to look for solutions to domestic policy challenges in other countries and from international organisations (for related studies see Deacon et al., 1997; Deacon, 2007; Orenstein, 2008; Yeates, 2008). Frequently, the focus of such studies has been on low-income, developing countries (for example,

Hein and Kohlmorgen, 2003), middle-income transition countries (for example, Deacon and Hulse, 1997; Orenstein, 2000, 2008) and international financial institutions like the World Bank (for example, Wogart, 2003). Less attention has been given to the fact that developed countries, such as many European countries, are also possibly subject to influences deriving from international organisations. An exception is the literature on the impact of the EU on national social and health policymaking (for example, Kleinmann, 2001; Koivusalo, 2005; Koivusalo and Ollila, 2008).

This chapter illustrates what such global social policies in the field of health care systems mean for a particular transition country. Drawing on the example of Poland, this chapter discusses how more general and abstract global ideas, concepts and prescriptions for health care systems are reflected in the work of global social policy actors focusing on a specific country, namely Poland; and in that way, potentially, have an impact on such national decisions as the structure and reform of the health care system. The international organisations addressed in previous chapters, such as the World Bank, WHO, the ILO and OECD, are actors with a worldwide reach, and, at the same time, have a specific history with regard to and specific activities targeted at European countries. The implications of such actors with regard to reforms of the Polish health care system, particularly at the beginning of the transition process, will be explored in this chapter. Before we examine the ideas and roles of external actors, though, we first turn to a general description of the Polish health care system.

7.2   The Polish health care system

Before the beginning of the transformation process, at the end of the 1980s, the Polish health care system was based on the so-called "Semashko model" (or Soviet model of health care). This was a strongly centralised, hierarchical system, mainly funded from the central public budget, and provided health care for the entire population.

Based on assessments of the various and significant shortcomings of that system, the health care system that was developed during the country's transformation process was a decentralised system of mandatory health insurance, with the responsibilities for administering the health care system distributed to subnational government levels, and it was re-established as part of the public administration reform process in the late 1990s. Health care system reform started quickly in the transformation process, and the main reform directions were decentralisation, allowing for private medical practice, and improving the infrastructure of public providers. The responsibility for providing health care services was distributed across different national and subnational policy levels. Between 1997 and 1999, the Law on Universal Health Insurance was introduced, establishing sickness funds to finance the population's health care provision.

The Constitution of the Republic of Poland (1997), in its Article 68, gives all citizens the right to equal access to health services. This implies that dependents of insured people, as well as unemployed people and others not able to make their own contributions to the system, are also included in health protection. It is impossible not to join the scheme.

The health care system is financed out of compulsory public health insurance. This system provides for almost universal coverage. At the beginning of the development of this new health care system, several health insurance funds were founded, but this resulted in unacceptable regional differences regarding the access and quality of health services. Therefore, from 2003 onwards, the main responsibility for financing health care in Poland has fallen upon the National Health Fund (NFZ) as the only health insurance institution.[1] The contributions are formally collected by the general social security institutions (ZUS and KRUS) (currently at 9 per cent of the calculation base), and then transferred to the NFZ.

Patients usually enter the system by contacting a primary care physician (a gatekeeper system). From there, they are referred to any specialist care needed. Changes of the primary care physician are possible twice a year. Upon referral, patients are free to choose any specialist outpatient clinic, and are put on a waiting list. From there, they might be referred to further specialist or hospital care. There is also free choice of hospital for elective surgery or further diagnostics; again this is organised by waiting lists.

The NFZ is responsible for financing health services, and makes contracts with public and non-public health service providers, supervised by the Ministry of Health. In order to avoid significant regional differences in health care provision, there are standardised contracting procedures. Given a number of imprecise regulations in the previous law, it was replaced in 2004 by the "Law on Health Care Services Financed from Public Sources". Following that, there were attempts to define negative and positive lists of health services to be covered by public financing.

Despite this central health financing institution providing health services for close to 100 per cent of the Polish population, it covers only about 65 per cent of total health care expenditure. Additional financing sources are the state budget, and private contributions. While access to health services is generally very broad and free of charge for the insured, for pharmaceuticals and a number of health resort services significant private contributions need to be made. This made up about 22 per cent of total health expenditure in 2009.

The regulation of the system is shared between the Ministry of Health, the NFZ and territorial subgovernments. In line with ideas discussed above, a key function of the state being to regulate (stewardship) the health care system, the Ministry of Health was gradually put into the role of the health policy regulator (developing previous functions involving funding and organising health care provision). Concrete health policy strategies and planning is laid down in the National Health Programme (currently for 2007–2015).[2] This programme is explicitly linked to the objective of reducing health inequalities, and to the work of the Commission on the Social Determinants of Health (for more on this Commission see Chapter 2, section 4; see also WHO Europe, 2012).

Overall, the Polish highly regulated health care system is performing rather well; despite persistence of the usual problems connected with health care systems. Not surprisingly, discussions about improving the health care system in Poland have continued over the past years, but with few significant changes to the system in place. Despite this, the country continues to struggle with issues such as public health care provider debt, and the quality and effectiveness of the system. At the same time, Poland was not one of the countries that was strongly hit by the global economic and financial crisis in 2008 and following years. Therefore the health care system was also untroubled by additional constraints that might have been caused by the crisis.

7.3   International organisations' engagement in Polish health care system reform

The World Bank's early missions regarding the Polish health care system

As could have been expected, particularly given our knowledge about external influences in the field of pension reform in Poland, with the World Bank being an important actor (Müller 2003; Orenstein 2005), we can detect early and intensive engagement of the World Bank with the Polish government on the question of how to make health system transition work from the beginning of the 1990s onwards.

Already at the very beginning of the 1990s, World Bank Health Sector and appraisal missions visited Poland for several weeks, and produced reports on the state and reform need of the country's health care system. In line with the general approach to economic reform that characterised the transition process, one important aspect was considered to be "improving health, strengthening the health sector's contribution to the social safety net, and containing upward pressure from the health sector on the state budget" (World Bank, 1992a: iv). The plan for reforming the Polish health care system was a project targeted at three designated regions that focused on health promotion, primary health care, health management and regional health services.

However, not only were particular World Bank projects had a conceptual impact on reforms, but the so-called World Bank Task Force on Health System Reform was also concerned with formulating the "strategic framework for a fundamental systemic reform in the health sector" in Poland. In the related World Bank report, we can read:

> [A]n improved health care system is critical to strengthening the safety net to protect poor and vulnerable population groups both during and after transition. [...] Upgrading health services to western standards is far beyond the financial resources that will be available to the health sector in the near future. The Government does not intend now to address all the issues in the health sector. Instead, it will address only those priorities that would have the greatest impact on improving health, increasing effectiveness and efficiency in the provision of health care and transferring some of

the responsibility for financing health care from the state budget to contributory social insurance.

(World Bank, 1992a: section 1.27)

The focus of the reported reform needs and the emphasis on particular steps was, unsurprisingly, concerned with financing. "Securing more adequate, stable and balanced revenues must be the cornerstone of the proposed health care reforms" (World Bank, 1992b). Accordingly, a need for strategic financial insurance to reduce overuse of services and contain costs was identified. The way forward was supposed to be regional resource allocation and budgeting.

In terms of the financing system, the focus was on contributory social insurance from early on. Regarding the provision of services, the first steps planned were to create so-called health care consortia, which would include all public and private providers. The initial plans and proposals supported by the World Bank were clearly focused on decentralisation.

This engagement by the World Bank, which by far extends the evaluation of project proposals and outcomes, suggests a direct involvement of World Bank staff with Polish decisionmakers in the course of the transition process. As reported in other studies, the World Bank also has the means to play a particularly influential role in health care system reforms. The concrete ideas that are fed into the national reform processes in the course of such missions may reflect the ideas expressed in major World Bank reports; however, they may also be highly dependent on the individuals who are part of the respective missions.

The WHO's multilevel structure for health care systems

Of course, a number of other global health actors matter and need to be studied concerning their possible impact and involvement in the Polish health care system development, even if the World Bank had an early and strong stake in the transition process. As shown in Chapter 2, section 4, WHO is *the* international organisation within the UN system, and it also builds an important point of reference in the context of the transformation countries in Central and Eastern Europe. While WHO's general approach has been characterised as "universal" in the sense of applying to all countries, European states are not only subject to that general approach, originating from WHO's headquarters. The WHO structure also includes six regional offices, one of them the European Regional Office, which is under-taking specific programmes and initiatives tailored to the 51 member states within that region. The specific roles of the WHO European regional office are, amongst others, to provide knowledge and infor-mation on various health topics; to promote the HFA policy in the European region, and provide tools to help countries achieve it; and to foster technical cooperation and build networks (WHO Europe, 1999: 5f.).

The World Health Report 2000 principles and models (see Chapter 2, section 4) have also been applied to the European region in publications by the WHO Regional Office for Europe, such as the HEALTH21: The Health for All policy framework of the WHO European Region (WHO Europe, 1999), and its Update in 2005 (WHO Europe, 2005); as well as in the European Health Report of 2002 (WHO Europe, 2002).

WHO, according to its overall work at the global level, provides models of health care systems, as well as discussing reform issues that are adjusted to the European region. These are often related to specific problems (such as demographic or financial challenges). In that sense, the WHO Regional Office runs a number of pro-grammes or projects directed to its member countries, for example the EUROHEALTH programme and programmes on Health Impact Assessment (HIA), on the quality of health care systems and on health care system organisation and management.[3] Specific groups of coun-tries within that region are addressed, as for example in the Health Development Action for South-Eastern Europe (SEE).[4]

A great emphasis in WHO work is on providing tools for assessing performance and to encourage member states to use them, to allow for comparison as well as mutual learning. Beyond the WHO's gen-eral target setting for the field of health care systems in its World Health Report 2000 (WHO, 2000) and its follow-up work (for exam-ple, Murray and Evans, 2003b), as well as its HEALTH21 framework for Europe. WHO further runs the HIA programme intended to "pro-vide tools and advice to Member states through building capacity for integrated impact assessments, and aims to increase the profile of health within other sectors' agenda by contributing with evidence on expected health benefits and risks".[5]

A central component of the WHO European Regional Office's work is the definition of the Health for All (HFA) policy frame-work for that specific group of countries as a response to the

WHA's call for "regional and national policies to be developed on the basis of the global policy" (WHO Europe, 1999: 3). This strategy for the European Region was formulated in a report entitled HEALTH21: The HFA policy framework for the WHO European Region:

> Both for western and eastern Europe, the only sensible way out of the present quandary is to ensure a more integrated health service system where PHC is equipped to solve all problems that can be effectively dealt with at that level, while hospital care is reserved for those that cannot.
>
> (WHO Europe, 1999: 119)

This framework was renewed in 2005 with the HFA policy framework for the WHO European Region: 2005 Update (WHO Europe, 2005), which particularly stressed the importance of values in the organisation of health care systems. This also includes a discussion on universal availability, universal accessibility, universal acceptability and quality improvement.

> In Europe, health systems can be described as having three essential goals – health gain, fairness and responsiveness. All three are in harmony with the Health for All concept. A health system that is driven by Health for All goals should also respond to the non-medical expectations of both individuals and society, for instance by safeguarding patient dignity, confidentiality and autonomy; respecting patient rights; being sensitive to specific needs and vulnerabilities of all population groups; and promoting social inclusion and poverty reduction.
>
> (WHO Europe, 2005: 18)

Concerning the European region, there is a particular focus on health *outcome* in health care provision, and a call for more (structurally and functionally) integrated systems (WHO Europe, 1999: 116ff.). Another important feature is the issue of *quality* of care, addressed for example in the Ljubljana Charter or the HEALTH21 framework. The HEALTH21 (WHO Europe, 1999: 130) framework also proposes more decentralisation in order to improve performance.

The tasks of designing an HFA-oriented community health policy, complete with targets and an action programme, and of executing, monitoring and evaluating its implementation, are vital components of the HFA approach that must be tackled on a properly planned basis by every local community in every Member State.

(WHO Europe, 1999: 160)

On financing, for the European region the Ljubljana Charter states that "health systems need to [...] ensure financing that will enable health care to be provided to all citizens in a sustainable way" (WHO Europe, 1996), and the HEALTH21 framework explains that "[m]easures should be taken to promote collective funding, whether by insurance or taxation to ensure solidarity and 'risk pooling'" (WHO Europe, 1999: 133). Adequate financial resources are said to be necessary; the amount should be affordable by the country in question and allow for health promotion and provision of effective and high-quality health care. For the European region, various sources of funding are identified, most often a mix; accompanied by a discussion about the advantages and disadvantages of different approaches and strategies.

The WHO, beginning with its World Health Report 2000, has strongly advocated the concept of stewardship, implying a strong role of the state in organising or regulating the health care system. For the European Region this is expressed as follows:

The health sector, under the governance of a ministry or department of health, has the primary objective of health improvement: it delivers health services, is responsible for health policy and management, and carries out activities oriented to both the individual citizen/patient and the community/population.

(WHO Europe, 1999)

Further, the importance of universal access according to need, plus targeting of vulnerable groups if necessary, is stressed. For the European region, in particular, it is pointed out that

Regardless of the main method of funding used, governments, as elected representatives of the people, have the responsibility of ensuring solidarity and universal access to health services, as well as of containing overall costs. Governments may have different positions, for instance as the main source of funds (in countries with taxation-based arrangements) or as the regulator of contributions (in countries with social insurance systems). In both cases however, their role in ensuring universal access and solidarity is crucial and should not be diminished.

(WHO Europe, 1999: 133)

Further important aspects especially for European health care systems are "to refocus on management of health services and measuring the time impact of different interventions" (WHO Europe, 1999: 130), citizen participation and information, and contracting arrangements between purchasers and providers. Concerning the performance of health care systems, it is proposed to decentralise health care management, increase competition, improve patient choice and focus on resource allocation (WHO Europe, 1999: 130).

Another development of European health strategies was provided by the WHO Regional Office for Europe through the Health 2020 report, which provides a policy framework and strategy for the European region, approved in 2012. More concretely, the Health 2020 strategy focuses on "health as a human right; whole-of-government and whole-of-society-approaches to equitable improvement in health; [and] strong and invigorated governance and leadership for health" (WHO Europe, 2013: 3). The aim is, in line with more global strategies (concretely mentioned is the WHO's Twelfth General Programme of Work (WHO, 2014), to develop new approaches and perspectives to realise universal health coverage. Regarding health systems it says: "Health 2020 acknowledges and celebrates the wide diversity of health systems and approaches across the European Region. It aims not to make national and local health systems uniform but to make them uniformly better" (WHO Europe, 2013: 9). The key problem identified regarding health care systems in Health 2020 is the relationship between the costs for health care and health outcome: "Many health systems fail to contain costs while financial pressures on them make getting the balance right for health and ensuring social protection ever harder" (WHO Europe, 2013: 12). Accordingly, priority area 3 of this strategy is entitled "Strengthening people-centred health systems, public health capacity and emergency preparedness, surveillance and response."

Overall, however, the strategy is not concrete, and does not seem to address the key health care system issues relevant to ensuring a comprehensive system of social protection. Instead we can read that we need "health care systems to give priority to disease prevention, foster continual quality improvement and integrate service delivery, ensure continuity of care, support self-care by patients and relocate care as close to home as is safe and cost-effective. The potential of personalized medicine needs to be assessed" (WHO Europe, 2013: 18–19).

Concerning the relationship between WHO and Poland more concretely, WHO Europe and Poland collaborate on the issue of health system financing reform, and Poland agreed on a biennial collaborative agreement (BCA) for 2012–2013. Among the priorities are the development and implementation of policies for health based on Health 2020; and health care systems strengthening. On the latter, the plan was to aim at

> health financing policies implemented in Poland to make progress towards, or sustain existing achievements of, universal health coverage, with attention to minimizing the negative effects of the financial crisis on the health sector and ensuring that financing and service delivery arrangements for priority personal and public health services are well aligned. Poland adopts and applies risk reduction strategies, norms and standards, which aim to enhance the quality and safety of health care services, through an integrated approach that focuses on the patient, the provider and the service.[6]

There have also been discussions about health issues between the WHO Europe and Poland in the context of tackling health inequalities. A related report was published in 2012 (WHO Europe, 2012), and made reference to the social determinants of health and the related "Closing the Gap" report (WHO CSDH, 2008). Among the recommendations of the report on Poland was the fair distribution of resources needed for health, and fair access to the opportunities available (WHO Europe, 2012: 92). In the same year as the report on inequalities in health was published, 2012, the WHO Regional Office for Europe also released the new Health Systems in Transition (HiT) (European Observatory on Health Systems and Policies, 2012).

We can see how general WHO concepts, those applied to countries in the European region and specific prescriptions on the Polish case provide a potential frame of reference for Polish health policymakers. Nevertheless, the processes we can observe in the case of the WHO are not comparable with the much earlier and stronger role the World Bank was able to play in the first years of transition.

OECD

Poland joined the OECD in 1997,[7] a couple of years into the country's transition process. A common feature of the OECD's (and WHO's) approaches for the European region or for more developed countries is the concentration on reform, and not primarily a basic model of health care systems, which is thanks to the fact that in most European countries more or less effective health care systems are in place. As the OECD's work on health is mostly focused on comparing health care systems, in contrast to promoting particular system or reform models, the basic approach is to study different member countries' models, reforms, solutions, problems in certain areas, compare them with each other and show advantages and drawbacks of different reform approaches or institutional arrangements. Doing that, the OECD provides, at least, a comparative contextualisation of the state of the Polish health care system. The interest is mainly in creating comparable data sets, which, of course, include an idea of specific functions of health care systems. This includes Poland, and we find regular data on the country's health indicators (and of course other policy fields and issues) that might affect the perceptions and assessments within the country of what works and what does not in national health policies.

Whether the OECD, by providing this kind of information, indirectly suggests particular models or reforms is a crucial, but difficult, question. The special interest in some of the OECD's work, for example, in issues such as private health insurance (PHI), could be an indicator for favouring private, market-driven health care systems. Taking a closer look at the Health Project report (OECD, 2004b), however, suggests a rather reluctant approach with regard to PHI (at least it is not openly promoted in or for countries (see Kaasch, 2010)). Usually, the OECD avoids norm-setting, in favour of comparing and presenting approaches employed in different countries.

The OECD, at least in the form of a working paper, has engaged with "Improving the Health-Care System in Poland" (Boulhol et al., 2012), related to the 2012 OECD Economic Review of Poland.[8] This paper gives a central role to the government in health systems issues, and suggests that required "extra resources should be financed by savings on other public expenditure items and possibly by additional revenues, which should be levied on tax bases that are least detrimental to economic performance, such as property and environmental taxes, and by cutting tax expenditure" (Boulhol et al., 2012: 5). More significant, the paper stresses, are thus the issues about access to care, along with persistent inequalities in Polish society. Part of the problem is said to be high levels of out-of-pocket expenditure, and the paper discusses ways to solve this. "[S]ome kind of graduated cost-sharing mechanisms" is considered, combined with a careful suggestion to learn from the Swedish model. Interestingly, here we find quite some space given to discussing the possibility of introducing PHI. As common for OECD papers, it is not a blank recommendation to introduce PHI, but more of a discussion about the advantages and disadvantages connected with PHI. Accordingly, the paper concludes: "Overall, PHI would likely contribute to improving health-care performance in Poland, but policy makers need to be aware of its possible downsides" (Boulhol et al., 2012: 24). However, it remains questionable if PHI should be the only option that deserves discussion.

In that way, and taking into account both the commonly broad trust in the value of OECD data and the processes of OECD governance, this organisation does have the potential to influence national thinking and reform steps in Polish health policies. However, at the moment, there does not seem to be a particularly strong OECD engagement with the Polish case.

ILO

Studying the ILO–Poland relationship concerning the country's health care system reform illustrates the limited scope and possibility of the ILO to engage in such reform processes. The ILO's website includes a page on Poland and social protection in health that gives a brief overview of the country's health care system.[9] In its recent strategic document on "Universal Health Protection" (ILO, 2014), there is at least a mention of the Polish case. As also discussed by other international organisations, the increasing health expenditure in Poland is also mentioned and discussed by the ILO. The short overview concludes by saying:

> The biggest challenge faced by Poland's health system today is its limited sources for financing social protection in health, which affects accessibility to services of adequate quality. Furthermore, the reliability of the health information system should be improved in order to ensure efficient and effective planning of human resources and infrastructure and improve the quality of care, in addition to minimizing the loss of financial resources.
>
> (ILO, 2014: 74)

It is unlikely that the ILO would be able to provide any more than general normative ideas about what health care systems should look like or be embedded in (in terms of social protection floors, for example). There is almost no means for direct application of ILO ideas to health care systems of specific member states.

European Union: The regional social policy context

Before concluding this study of the application of global health care system ideas in the case of Poland, the regional context needs to be considered as well (for regional social policy more generally, see Deacon et al., 2010). The EU has of course also formed an important context for Polish health care system reforms, and has appeared as an actor in the reform processes as well. The full impact of the EU accession process on the Polish health care system cannot be reflected in the context of this book, but a number of points may be useful in order to contextualise the global actors' involvement with Poland.

EU structural funds have been a key instrument in developing the new health care system in Poland (since the country joined the EU in 2004). The support was directed at infrastructure, occupational health and better quality management systems, amongst other things. Both Regional Operational Programmes and the European Social Fund gave significant contributions to support the system. In addition, the Polish health sector benefited from the European Economic Area grants, Norway grants, supporting health promotion and prevention programmes, as well as measures to improve access and quality, and reduce inequalities in health.

Furthermore, it was EU-sponsored health specialists who joined the World Bank appraisal mission that was involved in designing health care system reform in Poland in the early 1990s. Advice from that group of external experts may have equally carried EU perceptions and expectations of appropriate health care systems, as did those of the World Bank.

Some "transnational" activities have also happened, unsurprisingly, in collaboration between multi-level actors. An example of this is the WHO project "Support to health security, preparedness planning and crisis management in EU, EU accession and neighbouring (ENP) countries", which was supported by the European Commission Directorate-General for Health and Consumers. One output of this project was a report on Poland (2009).

Therefore, apart from concrete criteria to be met in order to join the EU, the European level of health policymaking has built a context for Polish health care system reform, as has been seen at a global level in this book.

Conclusions

This chapter has shown some of the international organisations' engagement regarding Polish health care system reform in transition. It is interesting to see that while the impact of external policy actors on the Polish pension system has been clearly shown in a number of studies, we know much less about the situation with regard to the Polish health care system. Following a political fight for competences and reform in the mid-1990s (Nelson, 2001: 256), the Polish health care system is now independent from pensions and the general social insurance system (providing income security for old age, disability, sickness and maternity). However, the reform process and the current shape of the Polish health care system can be seen as broadly fitting within the concepts and ideas about ideal health care system structures, as proposed by a number of international organisations and described in the previous chapters.

Nelson (2001) illustrates the different stories of pension and health care system developments in Poland and Hungary. He argues: "Given these complexities and characteristics, neoliberal economic concepts and approaches that have provided the paradigm for many of the institutional reforms in market-oriented structural adjustment may apply only partially and with substantial caveats in the health sector"

(Nelson, 2001: 260–261). This fits with the findings of the analysis of global ideas that has led to the conclusion that there is a lot of uncertainty involved in providing global prescriptions for health care systems. Furthermore, Nelson argues, quite in line with the argument developed here, that "pension reform is 'easier' than health-sector reform. Pension systems are much less complex administratively, nor do they generate large, powerfully organized providers' associations" (Nelson, 2001: 261). I have made a similar argument in Kaasch (2013).

As has been the case both for other social policy fields (particularly pensions) and for other former Communist countries, the World Bank has played a significant role in guiding and supporting the Polish health care system reform path from quite early on in the transition process. The decentralised system envisaged in the first years has, however, not prevented the country from recentralising its health care system a couple of years later (with the establishment of a single national insurance institution, the NFZ). The WHO's recent biennial agreement with Poland is rather focused on how to achieve universal coverage, and therefore speaks as much the current "common" language of global health policy, as the story of the World Bank's engagement tells us something about the 1990s.

The OECD, at the same time, remains true to itself in providing, on the one hand, data and well-balanced socio-economic discussions of the health care system situation and reform needs in Poland; and on the other hand, thinking over-proportionally about the provision of PHI for the country. The ILO, however, is very limited in its engagement, but clearly committed to a broader concept of social protection in the field of health.

The important context and role of the EU and the accession process shows that, beyond the engagement of global social policy actors, regional context and regional supranational bodies play an important role in the external shaping of national reform processes. Related arguments concerning the importance of regional social policies have been made in Deacon et al. (2010).

8
Conclusions: Multiple Actors, Uncertain Ideas, Nested Discourses

8.1 Introduction

This book has presented some of the key global social policy actors that frequently provide, in different ways, prescriptions for national health care systems. It has been structured as to first characterise activities and actors within the UN system, most prominently the WHO, the World Bank and the ILO. Chapter 3 considered the different but not necessarily less powerful roles of the OECD and WTO respectively. This rather traditional type of global social policy actor, the international (governmental) organisation, has been increasingly joined (and to some extent challenged) by other types of actor, such as the Global Fund to Fight AIDS, Tuberculosis and Malaria, and groups of countries (G7/8, G20, the BRICS) that have been discussed in chapters 4 and 5. Non-governmental actors, or CSOs, are plentiful in the field of global health more generally; however, concerning complex and explicit concepts of health care systems, Chapter 6 focused on one specific initiative, the Global Health Watch. Chapter 7 discussed the Polish health care system and external engagement in its reform by a number of these actors, showing how a number of international organisations have applied their ideas or concepts to specific prescriptions for this country in transition after the 1980s, and how global actors engage at a country level.

As part of the analytical framework used to analyse the ideas of global social and health policy actors, health care systems have been understood as part of the welfare state. This is related to comparative welfare state literature (most prominently, Esping-Andersen, 1990) and comparative health system studies (Moran, 1999, 2000). More specifically, the analysis followed a generalised health system model as developed by Grimmeisen and Rothgang (2004), and included questions on the context within which health systems are addressed, the goals and principles underlying the concepts, definitions of health systems, and the role of the state in different health system functions (provision, financing and regulation). While the issues with respect to provision and financing functions have been mainly on questions of public versus private, and centralised versus decentralised, the regulation function implied more specific relationships between service providers, financing parties and patients. The latter included issues related to the kind and mechanisms of coverage, the system of financing, service provider remuneration, access of providers to health markets, access of patients to service providers and the decision process about the benefit package (Grimmeisen and Rothgang, 2004).

It needs to be taken into account that the production of knowledge in the secretariats of international organisations is itself very much based on OECD countries' social policies. Surely, we can observe two things. First, there is a problematic use by global policy actors of Western models and solutions to problems in developing countries that have very different (social and health) needs. Second, there are various global health debates that go into the specific needs of developing countries, such as health issues related to malnutrition, maternal and infant mortality, malaria and other "tropical" diseases. One has to acknowledge that the ideas about health care system *models* are to some extent disconnected both in analytical means and in actual global social policy debates. This book, however, is not primarily concerned with such issues. It is focused on the "sender side" (global actors) and suggests only the relative or potential influence of actors. It is located at the global level in terms of an arena within which social policy debates take place, not about the appropriateness of these debates in capturing and responding to the real needs of countries.

The view of global social policy actors employed for the purpose of this book rests upon an understanding of international organisations (and other actors), a type of policy actor that – in its role and effect – is, on the one hand, more than just *one category* of idea provider, as expressed in the transfer literature; and, on the other hand, it is argued that policy diffusion is not necessarily as uncoordinated as suggested by Elkins and Simmons (2005: 39). Instead, these actors are understood as representing and providing a concrete location for the production, exchange and subsequent spread of ideas. International organisations, it is argued, have been created, define themselves and act as knowledge providers (on the role of international organisations in knowledge production see for example Stone, 2003; St Clair, 2006a), as well as platforms for exchange that facilitate policy diffusion or transfer between countries.

The argument rests upon the assumptions that, on the one hand, the foundation and existence of international agencies and initiatives is an expression for a desire of nation states to jointly react to health challenges; and that they are also a site of interaction between nation states. On the other hand, it is assumed that – once having emerged – those different actors build an independent system that develops ideas and activities that sometimes go beyond that first concrete task or original problem area. And once developed, their spread and the implementation of a model is not necessarily dependent on the existence of the specific original problem for which the solution was designed. The role of international organisations in transforming ideas and agendas has been pointed out by organisational theory (for example, Cyert and March, 1963; Olsen, 1997; Simmons and Martin, 2001).

The analysis reported in this book has shown that there have been a number of health system models put forward by international organisations. Comparing these ideas and concepts has revealed some differences, but much more important have been the similarities between the models. This final chapter is dedicated to drawing together some of the lines and implications of the findings presented, and discusses them within a broader frame of global social policy and governance.

8.2   Continuous, increasing but scattered awareness of health care systems in global arenas

Common ideas about health care systems

The idea of global health that guided the arguments in this book has been that of health and health policy having a significant transnational or global dimension in two ways On the one hand, health problems, including those that demand social protection and health system institutions, have transcended the arenas of national societies. As people move across national societies for various reasons, multiple connections, determinants and needs regarding health care systems arise. Not all of these can only be dealt with by national policymakers and institutions. On the other hand, national policymakers face similar problems and demands concerning health care systems, which gives rise to global comparative observations, possibly followed by policy learning or transfer, which again forms global health policy on national health care systems.

The analysis of a number of global health actors and their ideas about, and engagement in, national health care systems, reveals a number of characteristics of global ideas and discourses about health care systems. Concerning the content and processes of engaging with health care systems at, and from, the global level, one important finding is that, looking at global ideas about health systems, there seems to be a high degree of "common knowledge": functioning health care systems are considered to be indispensable, and they have to be inclusive, providing equal access to all those living in particular places. These are among the key messages to be found almost everywhere.

Interestingly, what we see are differences in the contexts within which health care systems are being addressed, and the goals or underlying principles in different organisations' approaches to health care systems. This includes, on the one hand, conceptions about human and social rights to health, and a concern about equity in health (Alma-Ata Declaration, Commission on the Social Determinants of Health); on the other hand, approaches dedicated to improving health and tackling poverty (also part of the WHO, but more importantly the World Bank and the Commission on Macroeconomic and Health; and also to some extent the ILO in connection with making a healthy workforce). The OECD provides a set of different ideas owing to its core group of mostly high-income countries and its working on a number of defined health system issues instead of approaching health systems as a whole. Accordingly, the definitions and conceptualisations of health systems also differ. Documents in the Alma-Ata tradition are rather interested in *levels* of the provision of care, while others are more focused on the *functions* of health systems (World Health Report, 2000 tradition).

Nevertheless, conclusions about appropriate and desirable health care systems with regard to their public-private and centralised-decentralised dimensions in provision and financing, as well as the proposed role of the state in regulatory relationships, do not differ that much between most of the actors that have been studied in this book, or differences are not explicit enough to discern. These similar ideas include the support of universal coverage (at least for basic care in a development context) and big risk pools (preferably public) in financing health care. However, global actors are careful in suggesting anything like a "one-size-fits-all" model. It is important to note that it is generally not a market-based model that is recommended. If the US health care system is mentioned, for example, in the documents, it is used as a bad example (for example, Roberts et al., 2008). A more comprehensive and systematic comparison both of the models of health care systems and of different global social policy fields has been provided by Kaasch (2013).

An interesting, though not very strong, difference between some of the models concerns the question of benefit packages. More concretely, the question of how a benefit package should be defined. Here, we can observe a difference between a process focus and a content focus. This means, for example, that a concept such as that of the WHO Commission on Macroeconomics and Health tries to define the content of, or the criteria for, defining an appropriate benefit package; while ideas from the ILO or in the Alma-Ata tradition always importantly contain reflections on the process of how to decide upon the benefit package (such as including particular groups of the population).

The actor constellations and advocacy coalitions that share a particular normative position, whether or not that extends to a comprehensive model, are not always, or not sufficiently, described by distinguishing between IFIs from UN social agencies. Instead what can be observed for global actors and ideas about health care systems involves a structure of broad synergies between the actors involved, with the exception of the IFC, on the one extreme, and Global Health Watch, on the other. The World Bank and the ILO differ from the Alma-Ata stream of ideas of the WHO, which concern the question of how to start building up health systems – with the aim of improving health as such or with the aim of (re)establishing equity. The World Bank and WHO (now with its World Health Report 2000 stream of ideas) go together on the analytical concepts of health system functions and their basic components. At the same time, we can observe how the OECD produces high-quality and even-handed work but only on very specific aspects of health systems, and avoids statements about the most desirable health policy. The role of the WTO, meanwhile, is very difficult to assess, as this organisation approaches the field with a completely different logic and does not provide explicit models of health systems and/or their functions. This situation makes it very difficult, if not impossible, to allocate actors and their ideas into clearly distinguishable health system advocacy coalitions (see also Kaasch, 2013).

Uncertainties in health care system prescriptions

At the same time as we can conclude a considerable degree of commonality between the models proposed, or prescriptions provided, by different global social policy actors concerning health care systems, what we can also see are fundamental gaps and a high degree of uncertainty regarding what works and what does not work for improving and developing health care systems.

Not only with regard to emergency situations, such as the Ebola outbreak in 2014, or an analysis of social determinants of health that call for comprehensive health care systems, what is a common feature in most of the reports analysed is a significant degree of "uncertainty" of what is the right thing to do about health care systems. The issue is not that there are no observable differences in and emphases on what could be appropriate, but they are not fundamental, as has been shown above; and often it is rather a complexity of issues illustrated than a convincing strategy on how to approach them comprehensively and in a sustainable way.

These complexities and the difficulties of associating health care system ideas produced and communicated by global actors with particular types of welfare state or health system arrangements has been partly explained by a perception of a lack of knowledge and lack of possession of a "best model" on the part of the international organisations. Current models or reform ideas can be at best characterised by adjectives such as *incomplete* or *fragmented*, and they tend to reflect a high level of uncertainty about "best health care systems". That is part of the reason why the ideas expressed by various actors do not add up to a comprehensive set of policy advice to approach health systems as a whole (see also Orenstein, 2008: 8f.).

Connected to this uncertainty, the analysis of health system ideas along public-private lines and degrees of (de)centralisation in the ideas proposed has not proved to be entirely feasible. Much of the consideration in related documents refers to advantages and disadvantages of different options without concluding on the best way. The most adequate summary of global ideas here would be that the state should be strengthened in the health sector without demonising private actors, but also not strongly promoting them. The only exception has been the IFC, which appears somewhat immune to otherwise shared ideas on priorities in health systems. However, the IFC's activities are a strategy for supporting private actors, not an attempt to formulate comprehensive concepts of health care systems.[1]

Historical shifts in focus on specific functions of health care systems

While historical shifts can be observed, these cannot only be understood as a shift from oppositional models towards more similarities (such as no more mention of user fees by the World Bank). It is rather, on the one hand, an increasing concern about health systems by all international organisations, accompanied by more intensive research activity, that apparently has led to similar conclusions in different organisations (supported by mutual exchange and networking activities (Lee and Goodman, 2002)). On the other hand, shifts have occurred in relation to the respective function of the health system in focus at a particular point of time. The focus seems to have shifted from provision to financing (WHO and World Bank) or financing to provision (OECD and ILO) and more recently to a particular emphasis on regulation. Some have interpreted this as a sign of the retreat of the state from financing and provision to a merely regulatory role. Looking at the findings of the analysis reported in this book, such a view cannot be fully supported. Regulatory concerns rather appear as a matter of strengthening the state's position in health care overall (in settings where there are perceived lacks), with considering private providers (and to a more limited degree also private insurers) to the extent that they contribute to efficient and quality care, but not at all at the expense of universal and equitable access.

Therefore, the analysis has shown that ideas about health systems are not characterised by significantly contested ideas that can be related to particular health systems or welfare state ideal types. The documents of different international organisations are not all the same – reflecting characteristics of the respective organisations such as original mandates or staff composition. The analysis has, however, not been designed to fully capture the "silences" that might lead to somewhat different results and conclusions. McCoy (2007) and the Global Health Watch 2 (2009) do this in relation to the World Bank ideas and strategies, while other literature (Banerji, 2002, 2006) has assessed the WHO's Commission on Macroeconomic and Health concept, also pointing to what it does not say or do. The WHO has been criticised for using the Commission on Macroeconomics and Health and its economic language to bid for legitimacy, but it could equally be understood as an attempt to translate social and health principles into an economic language. As shown by Heller and Hsiao (2007) and Roberts et al. (2008), the Commission on Macroeconomics and Health report indeed still provides a way of teaching economists some important features that characterise health policy that go beyond economic theory and need to be taken into account.

At the same time it is interesting to see how these different contexts and underlying principles, such as the aim of poverty reduction or striving towards more equality, still lead to rather similar models for the organisation of health systems. Apparently the common goal of universal access (to whatever broad package) leads to the same final models, while the desired route is still different. The World Bank would first target the poor through public funding of basic services, and once that is realised sees space for developing more sophisticated health systems (living with the unequal coverage for the transitional period); while the ILO would opt for micro-insurance systems to be merged into comprehensive systems in the future (thus accepting non-coverage for excluded groups for the transitional period).

Fluctuating global attention to health care systems

Another important issue is that, in terms of the emergence and changing of ideas, concepts or knowledge about national health care systems have varied over time: Despite permanent concern and awareness of the limitations of existing health care systems, the relative attention given to them at transnational policy levels is constantly changing – more than that, it shifts from one forum to another. This means either that all are concerned about health care systems, or all are more or less silent on the issue. The overall trend, though, is increasing and more permanent concern about health care systems by global social policy actors. That, however, only to a limited extent leads to more than changing terms, and a tremendous increase and decrease in attention to health care system over time; at the same time as more and more actors seem occasionally to raise their voice on health care systems.

At the same time, we see how fluid the concern about health care systems can be, related to the relative importance given to other policy fields at a particular point in time by the international community more broadly. The strong worries about the implications of climate change in particular – though of course important as such and critically linked with social policy and health policy in multiple ways – have the potential of turning attention away from health care systems. That is particularly worrying given the long-term implications of missing institutions of social and health protection in societies. Development and emergency measures, support and aid are of course crucial, but some of it can, and has to, be addressed with more enduring and permanent social policy arrangements and measures.

A recent example that shows the problem of not giving enough attention to health care systems becomes evident in the current Ebola crisis in a number of African countries. The obvious neglect in establishing and developing more comprehensive health care systems now forms part of the difficulties of handling the spread of a deadly disease. Numerous voices are now rising to claim that earlier chances to focus on health care systems in development aid have been neglected, and that there is a need now, at last, to take that issue more seriously.

Different ideas at the extreme ends

Despite the strong point made above about a high degree of shared ideas or common knowledge between global social policy actors on questions of health care systems, there are still some dividing lines between concepts, ideas and models brought forward by different global social policy actors. These are complex in nature and difficult to discern. Such differences between prescriptions can be identified in the details, such as the extent of public-private provision of health services; but not so much in terms of the basic goals of health care systems (for example, universal access) or a particular health care system model (for example, a social insurance system) by which universal coverage might be achieved best.

Nevertheless, the approach employed by the IFC significantly differs. It explicitly supports only private providers and private insurers without sufficiently taking into account more comprehensive concepts of, and concerns about, health care systems. This is even more astonishing as such ideas are provided by other parts of the World Bank Group. The IFC's ideas do not match those of the World Bank and appear not to be sufficiently coordinated with other World Bank activities.

At the other end of the spectrum, we find the very social ideas expressed by the Global Health Watch, that, to some extent, defines itself and gets its legitimacy by explicitly providing an alternative to common approaches.

The OECD is also somewhat different, but less in terms of the basic content than in terms of the context in which its activities are taking place (mainly high-income countries) and the related approach it takes to the guidance of national health systems. The OECD approach has been characterised as even-handed and of high quality. However, it needs to be taken into account that it is only partly comparable to the much more comprehensive agenda of other international organisations, both in terms of membership and approach to the topic.

8.3   Multiplicity, struggles of actors and dissemination strategies

Other important differences emerge when we consider structures and mechanisms of global actors that allow them to position themselves as important global health actors (that is, not necessarily linked to the specific ideas expressed). These differences become particularly clear when we consider the respective strategies and mechanisms available to a particular organisation for disseminating ideas and engaging with national health policymakers.

The number of global health actors – and not so much traditional health actors – is increasing without any doubt. It is now not only an issue for two or three major international organisations (the World Bank and WHO, to some extent together with the ILO). Instead, as health care systems matter in, and for, many other contexts, and cannot be separated from issues such as economic policies, food policies and so on, the activities around health care systems emerge in, or in changing coalitions of, organisations. In addition, they are increasingly sidelined by occasional attention paid to the issue by the major groups of countries (G7/8, G20, BRICS) and possibly others. To some extent, therefore, the organisations struggle over positions, and fulfil their role regarding health care systems based on different mandates and understandings of the meaning of health care systems within their respective roles in global social governance. The mandates may be direct or indirect (as has been illustrated with the potential impact of WTO activities on health care systems in Chapter 3). These differences also affect the legitimacy and power with which a particular organisation is able to disseminate health care system ideas.

It has been found that the different global health actors use rather similar means, but with differences in the quantity and quality of their use. The ILO probably comes closest to having some regulatory "power"; however, this is a fairly theoretical power that does not make it a particularly strong health actor. Health regulations by the WHO have not touched health systems in the sense studied in this book. However, it is still the most important norm-setting organisation on the scene. The World Bank, with comparatively least power to facilitate international health law, has, nevertheless, frequently been referred to as most powerful in influencing national health policy (through projects and conditional loans); but it is also a powerful source of numerous publications, and World Bank staff regularly teach a flagship course on health systems. The OECD is likely to gain increasing communicational power through its health data, comparative work and case studies on OECD health systems because of its reputation as a source of high-quality data and considered policy advice. In general, the main form of disseminating ideas has been the facilitation of exchange about health systems and thus non-coercive mechanisms of policy learning.

Judging the dissemination strategies that the actors use, this analysis has been limited by the fact that it mainly considered global-level processes, and thus the focus was mainly on the sender side of ideas (see Leisering, 2005). Thus, the strategies of international organisations were addressed without studying impact or complete transfer processes (even the chapter on Poland did not go any further than showing how international organisations approach, and relate to, health policies in the country). While notions of competition and unequal power distribution have implicitly characterised global social policy literature, conceptualising them and providing for analytical frameworks has not yet been undertaken in a sufficient way. Such perspectives on just one side of, or source within, transfer or diffusion processes have been difficult to analyse to a satisfying extent. A more meaningful discussion of dissemination strategies and the power of international organisations would certainly need to include analytical steps towards impact and effect of their activities. This could not be done within the scope of this book. The research reported here is, however, valid in the sense of mapping and discussing a *global* social policy process and scenery into detail that is commonly referred to in just one sentence as an assumption in other studies, without ever questioning the validity of related assumptions.

If we went a step further here, it would have to be considered that an important difference related to the power to spread ideas and influence national health policymaking concerns the different types of countries addressed by global policy actors. This can be seen by, in particular, looking at the World Bank's range of dissemination strategies, including conditional loans versus the OECD's careful approach to health policy models in the form of comparative discussions on the advantages and disadvantages of particular health reforms. This is not to suggest that the World Bank is not also influencing high-income countries with policy ideas (Orenstein, 2008) or that the OECD is only a point of reference to its own member states (Deacon and Kaasch, 2008). However, a careful distinction of the potential impact of different international organisations on different groups of countries (such as high-income, middle-income, low-income or transition countries) is a critical issue in understanding global social policy and the (potential) power of its actors. It would be worth taking into account such perspectives in further research into the field, thus looking at different implications and characterisations of such global social policy discourses, differentiating between different groups of countries and referring to their income levels as well as to regional affiliations.

This would probably also specify the different diffusion mechanisms as distinguished by a number of authors (for example, Orenstein, 2003; Elkins and Simmons, 2005; Braun and Gilardi, 2006). Events of policy learning might have a different character when taking place at an OECD ministerial meeting, at a World Bank flagship course or at a conference convened by the WHO.

Also, a better understanding of, and more careful distinction between, the different dimensions or mechanisms of global social policy would support a better account of different powers that are used to communicate ideas. Redistributional forms of global social policy connected to aid and/or conditionalities rather take coercive forms and often involve analyses of underlying notions or concepts of desirable social policy. The type of policy models analysed in this book are more about forms of learning and competitive or cooperative interdependence. Classifying mechanisms of global social policy and related forms of communication channels has important implications for generalising findings and characterising global social policy in general. This study, for example, has revealed that only a few actors are truly engaged in developing models for health systems, while others (most prominently the WTO) might have an important influence on the development of health systems using other global social policy mechanisms, namely forms of regulation or international law. It is important to improve our understanding of such mechanisms in order to avoid simple support or rejection of the involvement of particular actors, and not to support this with compilations of evidence that only speak for one interpretation of the matter.

It has further been shown that while international organisations do have a certain degree of autonomy and function independently as global social policy actors, they are nevertheless dependent on support from their member states, both concerning financing and legitimacy to act. The link to particular member states has not so much played a role in shaping concrete ideas or models, but it has been shown that different international organisations are in different ways empowered or constrained by their member states to act with regard to developing and communicating ideas on health systems. This includes the problem of particular images of, or unintended messages from, international organisations that influence communicational power. The example given has been the World Bank, which is always associated with the promotion of user fees, even though it has changed its position on this. Also, countries are engaged in decisions about the character and scope of international organisations' guidance of health systems; they ask for policy analyses and may or may not take up general or country-specific advice that has been produced in forms of studies and publications by international organisations. Accordingly, countries are not only *exposed* to global social policy actors.

8.4   Implications of different ways of engaging with concrete national cases

The example of Poland shows the parallel and, to some extent, inter-connected activities by a number of these organisations, namely the World Bank, WHO, OECD and ILO (and in addition the EU), concerning the reform and development of a national health care system.

The uncertainties around, and the lack of, comprehensive health care system models are replicated when it concerns national health reform, as exemplified with the Polish case. It is shown that social and health policy concerns are dealt with in a multilevel way, and studies should no longer be constrained to any one level. The differences, then, appear more indirect. For example, the OECD is mainly explor-ing the options of private health insurance for the Polish health care systems. The World Bank, in contrast, collaborated with the Polish government in the beginning of the transformation process (early 1990s), and during that time clearly supported decentralisation, a social health insurance system. WHO and ILO involvement is not particularly strong; however, in a regional social policy context, such as connected to EU accession processes, the WHO (Regional Office for Europe) seems to have been more involved.

8.5   The way forward

What does this mean for a better global health governance regard-ing the guidance of national health care systems? Starting with the CSO side, often considered to represent the "good" and "social" side of the actor spectrum, it has been shown that while indeed repre-senting an important (and social!) contributor of ideas on health care systems, the Global Health Watch runs the risk of mobilising forces on the ground through one-sided presentation of actors, by provid-ing inadequate information, favouring particular actors (for example, the WHO), while dismissing others (for example, the World Bank) that are also important global organisations which aim to improve health. Perhaps it is also a matter of having chosen a very complex

task that easily becomes too complex (even for international organisations with more staff and resources). It would be worth considering
whether it would not be better to partner with the other important
global health actors in order to strengthen health care systems by
providing knowledge about their functions and structures. Overall,
it is still a topic that suffers from too little knowledge and expertise.
As the contribution by Shaw (2007) shows, one should also be careful
with too much criticism of (particular) international organisations, as
that does not always and necessarily push them in the intended direction. For better global health governance on the matter, it would be
more productive to find a common denominator (such as the desire
to strengthen health care systems, or to improve the health of the
poor), and for specific actors to fulfil the respective roles that can be
best fulfilled by each of them. This does not exclude critically evaluating each other's actions; but would hopefully prevent the dismissal
of particular actors completely, and thereby providing incomplete
information.

The major international organisations involved, namely the WHO,
the World Bank, the ILO and the OECD, should now use the Ebola
outbreak to increase their work on health care systems and attempt
to get the issue back up on major political agendas. This should, of
course, be matched by and inform health-sector development aid,
such as that provided by the Global Fund.

While the world's major groups at times appear to be an important forum for these issues, it is unlikely they can serve as permanent
and reliable places in which to push the case for better health care
systems.

There is still much to learn about the dissemination strategies of
these different actors and their implications for national reforms of
health care systems; and it is hardly possible to come to conclusions
here as to whether they are used in competitive ways or rather characterise shared strategies. It is most certainly both at the same time. Still,
in the light of the conclusion that the policy models proposed do not
significantly differ, one has to ask if it matters who is most powerful
at the level studied in this book. This again speaks to more careful
distinctions between different forms of communicational power, and
the values of collaboration between strong global health actors.

Two issues remain to be mentioned. On the one hand, there is the
great attention given to the issue of climate change that currently

dominates global agendas (and shifts attention away from health), while at the same time, there are numerous connections between the fields of health care system and climate change policies. The other issue is the impact of the global economic and financial crisis on ideas about appropriate health care systems. Health care systems are complicated, abstract, hard to grasp – and so, after a time when even the attention to major global health problems has declined as a consequence of the global economic and financial crisis, health care systems are even less focused upon. It is questionable if the recent Ebola outbreak and the renewed call of some global health actors to, at last, focus on the importance of health care systems in tackling such disease outbreaks, will make a more fundamental change. In the absence of major controversies about the importance and meaning of health care systems among global health actors, the (common) challenge is to bring the topic to key global agendas, and keep it there.

Notes

1 Global Social Policy Actors and Health Care System Ideas

1. In the context of this book, "health system" and "health care system" are used synonymously.
2. http://www.ilo.org/addisababa/whats-new/WCMS_303405/lang--en/index. htm, accessed 20 November 2014.

2 UN Organisations: Health for All and All for Health Care Systems?

1. See http://www.un.org/aboutun/basicfacts/unorg.htm.
2. See http://www.norad.no/globalcampaign, accessed 29 November 2014.
3. http://sustainabledevelopment.un.org/focussdgs.html, accessed 29 November 2014.
4. The financial crisis and global health report of the high-level consulta-tion, Geneva 19 January 2009 http://apps.who.int/iris/bitstream/10665/ 70440/1/WHO_DGO_2009.1_eng.pdf?ua=1, accessed 29 November 2014.
5. http://www.oecd.org/newsroom/aid-to-developing-countries-rebounds-in -2013-to-reach-an-all-time-high.htm, accessed 29 November 2014.
6. See www.un.org/docs/ecosoc_background.html.
7. See http://www.un.org/docs/ecosoc/meetings/hl2002/.
8. See http://www.undp.org, accessed 29 November 2014.
9. See http://www.un.org/esa/desa/, accessed 29 November 2014.
10. The reports can be accessed at http://undesadspd.org/ReportontheWorld SocialSituation.aspx, accessed 29 November 2014.
11. http://www.who.int/whr/2010/en/index.html.
12. See jointlearningnetwork.org, accessed 29 November 2014.
13. See http://blogs.worldbank.org/developmenttalk/what-s-the-universal -health-coverage-push-really-about?cid=decresearch, accessed 29 November 2014.
14. See http://www.who.int/mediacentre/events/2012/wha65/en/, accessed 29 November 2014.
15. See http://hsr2012.healthsystemsresearch.org/, accessed 29 November 2014.
16. For more information on this topic, see also GSP Digest 12.2 following.
17. Though one of the major topics currently addressed by WHO and other organisations (owing to the focus and analytical framework of this book) this function is not taken into account.

18. For a discussion on the role of Jeffrey Sachs in global social governance, see Stubbs and Wedel (2015).
19. See www.who.int/social_determinants/strategy/enl.
20. Carissa Etienne moved to the Pan American Health Organization (PAHO) in 2013, after she had been elected Director of PAHO in September 2012.
21. http://go.worldbank.org/BTBAQHC530, accessed 27 November 2014.
22. This was accompanied by a Lancet series Alma-Ata: Rebirth and Revision.
23. Development Assistance for Health.
24. http://go.worldbank.org/1TEFJOO9F0, accessed 22 January 2015.
25. http://www.worldbank.org/en/topic/health/overview, accessed 24 April 2014.
26. See http://www.ifc.org/ifcext/che.nsf/Content/Strategy; original emphasis, accessed 9 July 2008.
27. See http://www.ifc.org/ifcext/che.nsf/content/strategy.
28. See http://www.ifc.org/ifcext/che.nsf/content/strategy.
29. This concern has also been raised in an interview with a World Bank staff member.
30. I quote here at some length in order to show several points already made in the previous chapter; that is, it is about *social* models, decentralised financing systems are regarded as a tool to enhance coverage (but not necessarily the final system to reach), private health insurance is not promoted and the US system does not serve as any kind of good example.
31. See http://www.worldbanktribunal.org/, accessed 29 November 2014.
32. Referring to Nelson, 2001.
33. See http://www.ifc.org/ifcext/che.nsf/Content/2007International Conference.
34. http://www.ifc.org/wps/wcm/connect/Industry_EXT_Content/IFC _External_Corporate_Site/Industries/Health+and+Education/, accessed 7 November 2014.
35. http://www.ifc.org/wps/wcm/connect/Industry_EXT_Content/IFC _External_Corporate_Site/Industries/Health+and+Education/Health +Sector/, accessed 7 November 2014.
36. The IMF at a Glance, Factsheet, May 2008, http://www.imf.org/external/ np/exr/facts/glance.htm, accessed 9 July 2008.
37. All quotes in this section from http://www.imf.org.
38. http://economistsview.typepad.com/economistsview/2006/02/martin _wolf_on_.html, accessed 29 November 2014.
39. http://web.worldbank.org/WBSITE/EXTERNAL/NEWS/0,,contentMDK: 21235530~pagePK:64257043~piPK:437376~theSitePK:4607,00.html, accessed 29 November 2014.
40. At the Philadelphia Meeting of the International Labour Conference the delegates adopted the Declaration of Philadelphia which was annexed to the Constitution and still represents the Charter of the aims and objectives of the ILO.
41. http://www.ilo.org/public/english/standards/relm/gb/docs/gb279/pdf/esp -7.pdf, accessed 29 November 2014.

42. See http://www.ilo.org/public/english/protection/secsoc/areas/policy/acti vity.htm, accessed 29 November 2014.
43. Now GIZ (Deutsche Gesellschaft für Internationale Zusammenarbeit – German Enterprise for International Cooperation).
44. http://www.socialhealthprotection.org, accessed 29 November 2014.
45. For example, Pathways to Improved Reproductive Health http://info. worldbank.org/etools/docs/library/122031/bangkokCD/ BangkokMarch05/Week1/1Monday/S3Pathways/Week1MondaySession3 .pdf; Health care systems http://info.worldbank.org/etools/docs/library/ 122031/bangkokCD/BangkokMarch05/Week1/2Tuesday/S2HealthSystem/ Week1TuesdaySession2.pdf, accessed 29 November 2014.

3 The OECD and the WTO: Outside the UN but Increasingly Important?

1. See OECD Health Update July 2005 https://www.oecd.org/dataoecd/10/57/ 35101765.pdf, accessed 29 June 2006.
2. However, first and foremost it is particular studies on the coordination of care; pharmaceutical pricing policies and innovation; disability trends and costs of care for older populations; health workforce and migra- tion; information and communication technologies; and the economics of prevention.
3. These are sickness funds, financed by compulsory, income-related contri- butions, which contract directly with independent providers of services, supplied free of charge to patients.
4. http://www.oecd.org/els/health-systems/characteristics.htm, accessed 16 November 2014.
5. See http://www.oecd.org/health/, accessed 29 November 2014.
6. See http://www.oecd.org/els/finalnewsrelease-meetingofhealthministers paris13–14may2004-towardshigh-performinghealthsystems.htm, accessed 29 November 2014.
7. According to one of my interviewees at the OECD.
8. Referring to Hoekman and Kostecki (1997).

4 The New Centres of Power? G8, G20 and the BRICS and Health Care Systems

1. http://japan.kantei.go.jp/summit/index_e.html, accessed 6 December 2014
2. http://www.mofa.go.jp/policy/economy/summit/2008/doc/doc080714 __en.html, accessed 6 December 2014.
3. http://www.jcie.org/researchpdfs/takemi/full.pdf.
4. http://www.g8italia2009.it/G8/Home/G8-G8_Layout_locale-11998821168 09_Summit.htm.
5. http://www.g8italia2009.it/static/G8_Allegato/G8_Health_Experts_Report _and_Accountability,0.pdf.

6. http://webarchive.nationalarchives.gov.uk/+/http:/www.dfid.gov.uk/
   Media-Room/News-Stories/2007/The-International-Health-Partnership
   -Launched-Today/, accessed 6 December 2014.
7. http://en.g8russia.ru/news/20140214/983221445.html, accessed 5
   December 2014.
8. http://www.brics5.co.za/about-brics/sectorial-declaration/health-ministers
   -meeting/beijing-declaration/, accessed 28 November 2014.
9. See http://brics6.itamaraty.gov.br/category-english/21-documents/186
   -communique-of-the-iii-meeting-of-health-ministers, http://www.brics.
   utoronto.ca/docs/140520-health.html, accessed 6 December 2014.
10. Labour 29, representing the interest of workers at the G20, see http://
    www.ituc-csi.org/l20?lang=en, accessed 6 December 2014.
11. G8/G20 Youth Network, representing young people's interests at the G20,
    see http://www.youthpolicy.org/library/documents/y8y20-summits-g8g20
    -youth-summits/, accessed 6 December 2014.
12. Civil Society 20, a platform for dialogue between political leaders and
    representatives of civil society organisations, see http://www.c20.org.au/
    about-c20/, accessed 6 December 2014.
13. See https://www.cigionline.org/events/roundtable-g8-and-g20-priorities
    -clashing-agendas-or-creative-tension, accessed 6 December 2014.
14. "Update 2009: Healthcare Under Stress", http://www.weforum.org/
    sessions/summary/update-2009-healthcare-under-stress.
15. See http://wsf2007.org.

5   The Global Fund to Fight AIDS, Tuberculosis and Malaria: A Hybrid Organisation as the Best Health Care System Actor?

1. http://www.theglobalfund.org/accesstolife/en/about/about-global-fund/,
   accessed 17 November 2014.
2. www.globalfund.org.
3. http://www.theglobalfund.org/en/replenishment/fourth/, accessed 17
   November 2014.
4. Health System Strengthening.
5. For background documentation of this report, see http://www.who.int/
   healthsystems/upcoming/en/index.html, accessed 28 November 2014.

6   Non-Governmental Organisations and Health Care System Ideas

1. http://www.gsdrc.org/go/displayandtype=documentandid=2802, accessed
   29 November 2014.
2. Referring to Fowler and Biekart.
3. www.ghwatch.org, accessed 29 November 2014.

4. The Global Health Watch 4 is about to be published at the time of writing. For information see www.ghwatch.org.
5. www.ghwatch.org/about; accessed 29 November 2014.
6. Tax Justice Network (2007) "Closing the Floodgates: Collecting Tax to Pay for Development". http://www.taxjustice.net/cms/upload/pdf/ Closing_the_Floodgates_-_1-FEB-2007.pdf, accessed 6 December 2014.
7. Gwatkin, D. (2003) "Free Government Health Services: Are They the Best Way to Reach the Poor?"
8. Brugha, R. (2008): "Global Health Initiatives and Public Health Policy", in: Heggenhougen, K. and Quah, S.R. (eds.), *International Encyclopedia of Public Health*. California: Academic Press.

7 The Polish Health Care System Under Global Scrutiny

1. The only link to the general social security system is that it falls to the Social Insurance Institution (Zakład Ubezpieczeń Społecznych (ZUS)) to collect all social and health insurance contributions.
2. Narodowy Program Zdrowia.
3. For all those programmes consult http://www.euro.who.int/.
4. http://www.euro.who.int/stabilitypact.
5. http://www.euro.who.int/healthimpact.
6. See http://www.euro.who.int/en/countries/poland/areas-of-work, and http://www.euro.who.int/en/health-topics/Health-systems/health-systems -financing/country-work/poland, accessed 17 November 2014.
7. http://www.oecd.org/poland/poland-and-oecd.htm, accessed 30 November 2014.
8. www.oecd.org/eco/surveys/Poland.
9. http://www.ilo.org/gateway/faces/home/polareas/socialsecurity/healthcare ?locale=ENandcountryCode=POLandtrack=nullandmpolicyId=9andpolicy Id=16andregionId=5and_adf.ctrl-state=vaedqni9n_46, accessed 17 November 2014.

8 Conclusions: Multiple Actors, Uncertain Ideas, Nested Discourses

1. However, this is still a matter for concern.

Bibliography

Abbott, Kenneth W. (2007) *Innovations in Global Health and the Global Governance System*. Vancouver: Wall Summer Institute (2007). Civil Society Organizations and Global Health Governance.

Abe, Shinzo (2013) 'Comment: Japan's Strategy for Global Health Diplomacy: Why It Matters', *The Lancet*, 382, 14 September 2013.

Alliance for Health Policy and Systems Research and WHO (2009) *Systems Thinking for Health System Strengthening*. Geneva: WHO. Available: http://whqlibdoc.who.int/publications/2009/9789241563895_eng.pdf (accessed 21 January 2015).

Armingeon, Klaus and Beyeler, Michelle (eds.) (2004) *The OECD and European Welfare States*. Cheltenham: Edward Elgar.

Banerji, Debabar (2002) 'Report of the WHO Commission on Macroeconomics and Health: A Critique', *International Journal of Health Services*, 32 (4): 733–754.

Barbosa da Silva, Jarvas, Keshav, Desiraju, Matsoso, Precious, Minghui, Ren and Salagay, Oleg (2014) 'BRICS Cooperation in Strategic Health Projects', *Bulletin of the WHO*, 92 (6): 388.

Barnes, Catherine (2005) 'Weaving the Web: Civil Society Roels in Working with Conflict and Building Peace', in Van Tongeren, P. (ed.), *People Building Peace 2, Successful Stories of Civil Society*. London: Lynne Rienner, pp. 7–24.

Barnett, Michael N. and Finnemore, Martha (1999) 'The Politics, Power, and Pathologies of International Organizations', *International Organisation*, 53 (4): 699–732.

Bartsch, Sonja (2003) 'Global Public-Private Partnerships in Health: Potentials and Limits', in Hein, W. and Kohlmorgen, L. (eds.), *Globalisation, Global Health Governance and National Health Politics in Developing Countries. An Exploration into the Dynamics of Interfaces*. Hamburg: Deutsches Übersee Institut, pp. 225–237.

Bartsch, Sonja (2005) *The Global Fund to Fight AIDS, Tuberculosis and Malaria: Establishment, Current Issues and Future Challenges*. Salzburg Seminar on the Governance of Health. OSI/Yale University/Temple University, Salzburg.

Bartsch, Sonja (2007) 'Global Public-Private Partnerships in Health: A Question of Accountability and Legitimacy'. Paper Prepared for the 2007 Wall Summer Institute for Research. Vancouver, 25–28 June 2007.

Bebbington, Anthony (2004) 'NGOs and Uneven Development: Geographies of Development Intervention', *Progress in Human Geography*, 28 (6): 725–745.

Bebbington, Anthony (2005) 'Donor-NGO Relations and Representation of Livelihood in Nongovernmental Aid Chains', *World Development*, 33 (6): 937–950.

Bello, Walden (2006) 'Afterthoughts: Critics Plan Offensive', *Global Policy Forum*, 27 April 2006.

Beyer, Joy A. De, Preker, Alexander S. and Feachem, Richard G. A. (2000) 'The Role of the World Bank in International Health: Renewed Commitment and Partnership', *Social Science and Medicine*, 50: 169–176.

Boulhol, Hervé, Sowa, Agnieszka, Golinowska, Stanislawa and Sicari, Patrizio (2012) Improving the Health-Care System in Poland, OECD Economics Department Working Papers, No. 957. Paris: OECD. Available: http://www.oecd-ilibrary.org/economics/improving-the-health-care-system-in-poland_5k9b7bn5qzvd-en (accessed 21 January 2015).

Braun, Dietmar and Gilardi, Fabrizio (2005) 'Taking "Galton's Problem" Seriously. Towards a Theory of Policy Diffusion', 46th Annual Convention of the International Studies Association (ISA), 1–5 March 2005, Hawaii.

Braun, Dietmar and Gilardi, Fabrizio (2006) 'Taking "Galton's Problem" Seriously. Towards a Theory of Policy Diffusion', *Journal of Theoretical Politics*, 18 (3): 298–322.

Bretton Woods Project (2011) 'IMF's European Austerity Drive Goes on, Despite Failures and Protests', *Bretton Woods Update Issue* 76, 13 June 2011.

Brolan, Claire E., Hill, Jonas and Hill, Peter S. (2013) 'Global Governance for Universal Health Coverage: Could a Framework Convention on Global Health Hold It Together?' *Global Health Governance*, 6 (2): 1–11.

Brooks, Sarah M. (2005) 'Interdependent and Domestic Foundations of Policy Change: The Diffusion of Pension Privatization Around the World', *International Studies Quarterly*, 49: 273–294.

Brooks, Sarah M. (2007) 'When Does Diffusion Matter? Explaining the Spread of Structural Pension Reforms Across Nations', *Journal of Politics*, 3: 701–715.

Brugha, Ruairí and Zwi, Anthony B. (2002) 'Global Approaches to Private Sector Provision: Where Is the Evidence', in Lee, K., Buse, K. and Fustukian, S. (eds.), *Health Policy in a Globalising World*. Cambridge: Cambridge University Press, pp. 63–77.

Brunet-Jailly, Joseph (1999) 'Has the World Bank a Strategy on Health', *International Social Science Journal*, 51 (161): 347–361.

Buse, Kent, Hein, Wolfgang and Drager, Nick (eds.) (2009) *Making Sense of Global Health Governance. A Policy Perspective*. Basingstoke and New York: Palgrave Macmillan.

Buse, Kent and Walt, G. (2000) 'Global Public-Private Partnerships: Part II – What Are the Health Issues for Global Governance?' *Bulletin of the World Health Organization*, 78 (5): 699–709.

Buse, Kent and Walt, Gill (2002) 'Globalisation and Multilateral Public-Private Health Partnerships: Issues for Health Policy', in Lee, K., Buse, K. and Fustukian, S. (eds.), *Health Policy in a Globalising World*. Cambridge: Cambridge University Press, pp. 41–62.

Castells, M. (2000) *The Rise of the Network Society: The Information Age: Economy, Society and Culture*. Oxford: Blackwell.

Centre For Global Development (2007) *Does the IMF Constrain Health Spending in Poor Countries? Evidence and an Agenda for Action*. Washington,

DC: Center for Global Development. Available: http://www.cgdev.org/ content/publications/detail/14103; (accessed 9 July 2008).

Chan, Margaret (2011) *WHO Director-General Addresses First Meeting of BRICS Health Ministers. 11th July 2011.* Beijing: WHO. Available: http://www.who .int/dg/speeches/2011/BRICS_20110711/en/ (accessed 4 December 2014).

Chand, Sudeep, Morrison, J. Stephen, Piot, Peter and Heymann, David L. (2010) 'From G8 to G20, Is Health Next in Line?' *The Lancet* (23 June 2010).

Clark, J. (1991) *Democratizing Development: The Role of Voluntary Organizations.* London: Earthscan. Constitution of the World Health Organisation. Available: http://www.who.int/governance/eb/who_constitution_en .pdf (accessed 21 January 2015).

Cooper, Andrew F., Kirton, John J. and Schrecker, Ted (eds.) (2007) *Governing Global Health. Challenge, Response, Innovation.* Aldershot: Ashgate.

Cyert, R. M. and March, James G. (1963) *A Behavioral Theory of the Firm.* Englewood Cliffs: Prentice Hall.

Dagmar (2003) 'The Impact of the World Bank on Health Care Reform in Transitional Economies', *Politicka Misao*, XL (5): 30–51.

Deacon, Bob (2003) 'Global Social Governance Reform: From Institutions and Policies to Networks, Projects and Partnerships', in Deacon, B., Ollila, E., Koivusalo, M. and Stubbs, P. (eds.), *Global Social Governance. Themes and Prospects.* Helsinki: Ministry for Foreign Affairs of Finland. Department for International Development Cooperation, pp. 11–35.

Deacon, Bob (2007) *Global Social Policy and Governance.* London: Sage.

Deacon, Bob (2008) 'Global and Regional Social Governance', in Yeates, N. (ed.), *Understanding Global Social Policy.* Bristol: The Policy Press, pp. 25–48.

Deacon, Bob (2013) *Global Social Policy in the Making.* Bristol: Policy Press.

Deacon, Bob (2014) 'Towards a Transformative Global Social Policy?' in Kaasch, A. and Stubbs, P. (eds.), *Transformations in Global and Regional Social Policies.* Basingstoke: Palgrave Macmillan, pp. 201–217.

Deacon, B. and Hulse, M. (1997) 'The Making of Post-Communist Social Policy: The Role of International Agencies', *Journal of Social Policy*, 26: 43–62.

Deacon, Bob, Hulse, Michelle and Stubbs, Paul (1997) *Global Social Policy: International Organizations and the Future of Welfare.* London: SAGE.

Deacon, Bob and Kaasch, Alexandra (2008) 'The OECD's Social and Health Policy: Neo-Liberal Stalking Horse or Balancer of Social and Economic Objectives', in Mahon, R. and Mcbride, S. (eds.), *The OECD and Global Governance.* Seattle: UBC Press, pp. 226–241.

Deacon, Bob, Macovei, Maria Cristina, Langehove, Luk Van and Yeates, Nicola (eds.) (2010) *World-Regional Social Poland and Global Governance.* New Research and Policy Agendas in Africa, Asia, Europe and Latin America. London: Routledge.

Delisle, Hélène, Hatcher Roberts, Janet, Munro, Michelle, Jones, Lori and Gyorkos, Theresa W. (2005) 'The Role of NGOs in Global Health Research for Development', *Health Research Policy and Systems*, 3 (3).

Docteur, Elizabeth and Oxley, Howard (2003) *Health-Care Systems: Lessons from the Reform Experience*. Paris: OECD.

Dodgson, Richard and Lee, Kelley (2002) 'Global Health Governance: A Conceptual Review', in Wilkinson, R. and Hughes, S. (eds.), *Global Governance: Critical Perspectives*. London and New York: Routledge, pp. 92–110.

Dolowitz, D., Greenwold, S. and Marsh, D. (1999) 'Policy Transfer: Something Old, Something New, Something Borrowed, but Why Red, White and Blue?' *Parliamentary Affairs*, 52 (4): 719–730.

Dolowitz, David P. and Marsh, David (2000) 'Learning from Abroad: The Role of Policy Transfer in Contemporary Policy-Making', *Governance: An International Journal of Policy and Administration*, 13 (1): 5–24.

Drabek, Anne Gordon (1987) 'Development Alternatives: The Challenge for NGOs – An Overview of the Issues', *World Development*, 15 (Supplement): ix–xv.

Dräger, Sigrid, Gedik, Gulin and Dal Poz, Mario R. (2006) 'Health Workforce Issues and the Global Fund to Fight AIDS, Tuberculosis and Malaria: An Analytical Review', *Human Resources for Health*, 4 (23).

Einhorn, Jessica (2001) 'The World Bank's Mission Creep', *Foreign Affairs*, 80 (5): 22–35.

Elkins, Zachary and Simmons, Beth (2005) 'On Waves, Clusters, and Diffusion: A Conceptual Framework', *The Annals of the American Academy of Political and Social Science*, 598: 33–51.

Ervik, Rune (2005) 'Battle of Future Pensions: Global Accounting Tools, International Organizations and Pension Reforms', *Global Social Policy*, 5 (1): 29–54.

European Observatory on Health Systems and Policies (2012) Health Systems in Transition, Poland, Health System Review 2011; 13 (8). Available: http://www.euro.who.int/__data/assets/pdf_file/0018/163053/e96443.pdf?ua=1 (accessed 21 January 2015).

Evans, M. and Davies, J. (1999) 'Understanding Policy Transfer: A Multi-Level, Multi-Disciplinary Perspective', *Public Administration*, 77 361–385.

Farnsworth, Kevin (2005) 'Promoting Business-Centred Welfare: International and European Perspectives on Social Policy', *Journal of European Social Policy*, 15 (1): 65–80.

Farrington, J. and Bebbington, A. (1993) *Reluctant Partners? NGOs, the State and Sustainable Agricultural Development*. London: Routledge.

Field, M. G. (1973) 'The Concept of the "Health System" at the Macrosociological Level', *Social Science and Medicine*, 7 (10): 763–785.

Florini, Ann M. (2000a) 'Lessons Learned', in Florini, A. M. (ed.), *The Third Force: The Rise of Transnational Civil Society*. Tokyo, Washington, DC: Japan Center for International Exchange, Carnegie Endowment for International Peace, pp. 211–240.

Florini, Ann M. (ed.) (2000b) *The Third Force. The Rise of Transnational Civil Society*, Tokyo, Washington, DC: Japan Center for International Exchange and Carnegie Endowment for International Peace.

Fox, Jonathan and Brown, L. David (1998) *The Struggle for Accountability: The World Bank, NGOs, and Grassroot Movements*. Cambridge, MA: The MIT Press.

GASPP Team (2005) 'Copenhagen Social Summit Ten Years On: The Need for Effective Social Policies Nationally, Regionally and Globally', *GASPP Policy Brief*, 6, pp. 1–8.

Gilmore, Anna, Collin, Jeff and Townsend, Joy (2007) 'Transnational Tobacco Company Influence on Tax Policy During Privatization of a State Monopoly: British American Tobacco and Uzbekistan', *American Journal of Public Health*, 97 (11): 2001–2009.

Global Health Strategies Initiative (2012) Shifting Paradigm. How the BRICS Are Reshaping Global Health and Development. Available: http://www.g20civil.com/documents/brics/ghsi_brics_report.pdf (accessed 21 January 2015).

Global Health Watch (2005) *2005–2006. An Alternative World Health Report*. London, New York: Zed Books.

Global Health Watch (2009) *An Alternative World Health Report*. London: Zed Books.

Global Health Watch 3 (2011) *An Alternative World Health Report*. London: Zed Books.

Gottret, Pablo and Schieber, George (2006) *Health Financing Revisited. A Practitioner's Guide*. Washington, DC: The World Bank.

Grimmeisen, Simone and Rothgang, Heinz (2004) *The Changing Role of the State in Europe's Health Care Systems*. Paper presented at the Annual ESPAnet Conference. University of Oxford.

G7 Foreign Ministers (2014) G7 *Foreign Ministers' Joint Statement on Ebola. 25th September 2014*. New York: G7. Available: http://iipdigital.usembassy.gov/st/english/texttrans/2014/09/20140925308907.html?CP.rss=true#axzz3KkYqAm3x (accessed December 2014).

G8 (2002) *G8 Africa Action Plan*. Kananaskis Summit, 27th June 2002. Kananaskis: G8. Available: http://www.g8.utoronto.ca/summit/2002kananaskis/africaplan.html (accessed 3 December 2014).

G8 Health Experts (2008a) *G8 Health Experts Meeting. 14th–15th February 2008. United Nations University*. Tokyo: G8 Health Experts. Available: http://www.g8.utoronto.ca/healthmins/health080215.html (accessed 3 December 2014).

G8 Health Experts (2008b) *Toyako Framework for Action on Global Health. Report of the G8 Health Experts Group. 8th July 2008*. Toyako: G8 Health Experts. Available: http://www.mofa.go.jp/policy/economy/summit/2008/doc/pdf/0708_09_en.pdf (accessed 3 December 2014).

Gwatkin, Davidson R., Wagstaff, Adam and Yazbeck, Abdo S. (eds.) (2005) *Reaching the Poor with Health, Nutrition and Population Services. What Works, What Doesn't, and Why*. Washington, DC: World Bank.

Haas, Peter M. (1992) 'Introduction: Epistemic Communities and International Policy Coordination', *International Organization*, 46 (1): 1–35.

Häkkinen, Unto and Ollila, Eeva (2000) *The World Health Report 2000. What Does It Tell Us about Health Systems? Analyses from Finish Experts*. Finland: Stakes, pp. 9–16.

Hanefeld, Johanna (2011) 'Global Fund to Fight AIDS, Tuberculosis and Malaria', in Hale, T. and Held, D. (eds.), *Handbook of Transnational Governance. Institutions and Innovations*. Cambridge: Polity Press, pp. 161–165.

Harmer, Andrew, Xiao, Yina and Tediosi, Fabricio (2013) ' "BRICS Without Straw"? A Systematic Literature Review of Newly Emerging Economies' Influence in Global Health', *Globalization and Health*, 9 (15).

Hein, Wolfgang, Bartsch, Sonja and Kohlmorgen, Lars (eds.) (2007) *Global Health Governance and the Fight Against HIV/AIDS*. Basingstoke and New York: Palgrave Macmillan.

Hein, Wolfgang and Kohlmorgen, Lars (eds.) (2003) *Globalisation, Global Health Governance and National Health Politics in Developing Countries. An Exploration into the Dynamics of Interfaces*. Hamburg: Deutsches Übersee Institut.

Hein, Wolfgang and Kohlmorgen, Lars (2008) 'Global Health Governance: Conflicts on Global Social Rights', *Global Social Policy*, 8 (1): 80–108.

Held, David and Mcgrew, Anthony (2002) 'Introduction', in Held, D. and McGrew, A. (eds.), *Governing Globalisation. Power Authority and Global Governance*. Cambridge: Polity Press, pp. 1–21.

Her Majesty's Government (2008) *Health Is Global. A UK Government Strategy 2008–2013*. London: Her Majesty's Government. Available: http://www.ghd-net.org/sites/default/files/UK%20gov.pdf (accessed 4 December 2014).

Hoekman, B. and Kostecki, M. (1997) *The Political Economy of the World Trading System*. Oxford: Oxford University Press.

Holden, Chris (2003) *The Global Healthcare Complex: Extent and Regulatory Issues*. Bristol: Policy and Politics in a Globalizing World. Conference.

Holden, Chris (2005) 'Privatization and Trade in Health Services: A Review of Evidence', *International Journal of Health Services*, 35 (4): 675–689.

Hsiao, William and Heller, Peter S. (2007) *What Should Macroeconomists Know about Health Care Policy?* Washington, DC: IMF.

ILO (2001) Social Security: *A New Consensus*. Geneva: ILO. Available: http://www.ilo.org/wcmsp5/groups/public/---ed_protect/—soc_sec/documents/publication/wcms_209311.pdf (accessed 6 December 2014).

ILO (2010) *World Social Security Report 2010/2011. Providing Coverage in Times of Crisis and Beyond*. Geneva: ILO.

ILO (2014) *Universal Health Protection: Progress to Date and the Way Forward*. Geneva: ILO. Available: http://www.ilo.org/wcmsp5/groups/public/---ed_protect/---soc_sec/documents/publication/wcms_305947.pdf.

ILO, GTZ and WHO (2006) *Berlin Recommendation for Action – Final Version – 3 July 2006*. International Conference on Social Insurance in Developing Countries, 05–07 December 2005. Berlin.

ILO and ISSA (1997) *Social Health Insurance*. Geneva: ILO.

ILO Social Security Department (2007) *Social Health Protection. An ILO Strategy Towards Universal Access to Health Care. A Consultation*. Geneva: ILO. Available: http://www.ilo.org/public/english/protection/secsoc/downloads/healthpolicy.pdf.

ILO Social Security Department (2008) *Can Low-Income Countries Afford Basic Social Security?* Geneva: ILO.

ILO Step (2005) *Health Micro-Insurance Schemes: Feasibility Study Guide. Vol. 1: Procedure.* Geneva: ILO.

Initiative, Global Health Strategies (2012) Shifting Paradigm. How the BRICS are Reshaping Global Health and Development. Available: http://www.g20civil.com/documents/brics/ghsi_brics_report.pdf.

International Labour Office (2000) *World Labour Report 2000: Income Security and Social Protection in a Changing World.* Geneva: ILO.

International Labour Office (2001) *Social Security: A New Consensus.* Geneva: ILO.

International Labour Office (2005) *Governing Body. Committee on Employment and Social Policy. GB.294/ESP/4, 294th Session.* Geneva: ILO.

IPCC (2007) Climate Change 2007: Synbook Report. Valencia: IPCC. Available: http://www.ipcc.ch/pdf/assessment-report/ar4/syr/ar4_syr.pdf (accessed 3 December 2014).

Jha, Prabhat and Chaloupka, Frank J. (2000) 'The Economics of Global Tobacco Control', *British Medical Journal,* 321: 358–361.

Jordan, Lisa and Van Tuijl, Peter (2000) 'Political Responsibility in Transnational NGO Advocacy', *World Development,* 28 (12): 2051–2065.

Kaasch, Alexandra (2007) Overlapping and Competing Agencies in Global Health Governance. WHO, World Bank, and OECD in the Guidance of National Health Care Systems. Paper Prepared for the ISA RC19 Annual Academic Conference, Florence, 6–8 September 2007.

Kaasch, Alexandra (2010) 'A New Global Health Actor? The OECD's Careful Guidance of National Health Care Systems', in Martens, K. and Jakobi, A. (eds.), *Mechanisms of OECD Governance – International Incentives for National Policy Making?* Oxford: Oxford University Press, pp. 180–197.

Kaasch, Alexandra (2013) Contesting Contestation: Global Social Policy Prescriptions on Pensions and Health Systems. Global Social Policy 13.1, pp. 45–65.

Kaasch, Alexandra (forthcoming) 'Conceptualising Global Social Rights', in Fischer-Lescano, A. and Möller, K. (eds.), *Transnationale Sozialen Rechte.*

Kaasch, Alexandra and Stubbs, Paul (eds) (2014) Transformations in Global and Regional Social Policies. Basingstoke: Palgrave Macmillan.

Kaasch, Alexandra and Martens, Kerstin (eds.) (2015) *Actors and Agency in Global Social Governance.* Oxford: Oxford University Press.

Kaldor, Mary (2003) *Global Civil Society: An Answer to War.* Cambridge: Polity Press.

Kapur, Devesh (1998) 'The IMF: A Cure or a Curse', *Foreign Policy,* 111: 114–129.

Kapur, Devesh and McHale, John (2005) *Give Us Your Best and Brightest: The Global Hunt for Talent and Its Impact on the Developing World.* Washington, DC: Center for Global Development.

Kaul, Inge, Conceicao, Pedro, Le Gouvlen, Katell and Mendoza, Ronald R. (eds.) (2003) *Providing Global Public Goods. Managing Globalization.* New York: Oxford University Press.

Kaul, Inge, Grunberg, Isabelle and Stern, Marc A. (eds.) (1999) *Global Public Goods: International Cooperation in the 21st Century*. New York: Oxford University Press.

Kay, Adrian and Williams, Owain David (eds.) (2009) *Global Health Governance. Crisis, Institutions and Political Economy*. Basingstoke and New York: Palgrave Macmillan.

Keck, M. and Sikkink, K. (1998) *Activists Beyond Borders: Advocacy Networks in International Politics*. Ithaca, NY: Cornell University Press.

Keefe, Tania J. and Zacher, Mark W. (2008) *The Politics of Global Health Governance*. Basingstoke and New York: Palgrave Macmillan.

Keohane, Robert O. and Nye, Joseph S. (2000) 'Introduction', in Nye, J. S. and Donahue, J. D. (eds.), *Governance in a Globalizing World*. Washington, DC: Brookings Institutions, pp. 1–41

Kickbusch, Ilona (2000) 'The Development of International Health Policies – Accountability Intact?' *Social Science and Medicine*, 51: 979–989.

Kickbusch, Ilona (2003) 'Global Health Governance: Some Theoretical Considerations on the New Political Space', in Lee, K. (ed.), *Health Impacts of Globalization. Towards Global Governance*. Basingstoke and New York: Palgrave Macmillan, pp. 192–203.

Kickbusch, Ilona (2004) 'Action on Global Health: Addressing Global Health Governance Challenges', *Public Health*, 119: 969–973.

Ki-Moon, Ban (2011) 'Remarks to the General Assembly Meeting on the Prevention and Control of Non-Communicable Diseases', *UN News Centre*, 19 September 2011.

Kirton, John J., Kulik, Julia and Bracht, Caroline (2014) 'Generating Global Health Governance Through BRICS Summitry', *Contemporary Politics*, 20 (2): 146–162.

Kleinmann, Mark (2001) *A European Welfare State? European Union Social Policy in Context*. Basingstoke: Palgrave Macmillan.

Koivusalo, Meri (1999) *World Trade Organization and Trade-Creep in Health and Social Policies*. Helsinki: Stakes.

Koivusalo, Meri (2003a) 'Assessing the Health Policy Implications of WTO Trade and Investment Agreements', in Lee, K. (ed.), *Health Impacts of Globalization. Towards Global Governance*. Basingstoke and New York: Palgrave Macmillan, pp. 161–176.

Koivusalo, Meri (2003b) 'Global Governance, Trade and Health Policy', in Hein, W. and Kohlmorgen, L. (eds.), *Globalisation, Global Health Governance and National Health Politics in Developing Countries. An Exploration into the Dynamics of Interfaces*. Hamburg: Deutsches Übersee Institut, pp. 203–223.

Koivusalo, Meri (2003c) 'The Impact of WTO Agreements on Health and Development Policies', *GASPP Policy Brief*, 3 (January 2003).

Koivusalo, Meri (2005d) 'The Future of European Health Policies', *International Journal of Health Services*, 35 (2): 325–342.

Koivusalo, Meri and Mackintosh, Maureen (2004) 'Health Systems and Commercialisation. In Search of Good Sense'. Prepared for the UNRISD

International Conference on Commercialisation of Health Care: Global and Local Dynamics and Policy Responses DRAFT, 2004 Geneva. UNRISD.

Koivusalo, Meri and Ollila, Eeva (1997) *Making a Healthy World*. Helsinki: STAKES.

Koivusalo, Meri and Ollila, Eeva (2008) 'Global Health Policy', in Yeates, N. (ed.), *Understanding Global Social Policy*. Bristol: The Policy Press, pp. 149–177.

Kruse, Johannes and Martens, Kerstin (2015) 'NGOs as Actors in Global Social Governance', in Kaasch, A. and Martens, K. (eds.), *Actors and Agency in Global Social Governance*. Oxford: Oxford University Press.

Kulik, Julia (2011) *Russia's Global Health Governance Gap: A Strategy for Summit Success*. Washington, DC: Centre for Strategic and International Studies, available: http://www.ghdp.utoronto.ca/pubs/kulik-russia.pdf.

Lee, Kelley (ed.) (2003) *Health Impacts of Globalization. Towards Global Governance*. Basingstoke: Palgrave Macmillan.

Lee, Kelley (2007) *The Role of CSOs in Intergovernmental Health Organisations: Contributions to Global Health Governance*. Wall Summer Institute 2007. Civil Society Organisations and Global Health Governance. Vancouver, 25–28 June 2007.

Lee, Kelley (2009) *The World Health Organization (WHO)*. Oxford, New York: Routledge.

Lee, Kelley, Buse, Kent and Fustukian, Suzanne (eds.) (2002) *Health Policy in a Globalising World*. Cambridge: Cambridge University Press.

Lee, Kelley and Goodman, Hilary (2002) 'Global Policy Networks: The Propagation of Health Care Financing Reform Since the 1980s', in Lee, K., Buse, K. and Fustukian, S. (eds.), *Health Policy in a Globalising World*. Cambridge: Cambridge University Press, pp. 97–119.

Leisering, Lutz (2005) 'Social Policy Learning und Wissensdiffusion in einer globalisierten Welt (Social Policy Learning and Knowledge Diffusion in a Globalised World)', in Becker, U., Zheng, G. and Darimont, B. (eds.), *Grundfragen und Organisation der Sozialversicherung in China und Deutschland (Basic Questions and Organisation of Social Insurance in China and Germany)*. Baden-Baden: Nomos, pp. 73–95.

Leisering, Lutz (2007) 'Gibt es einen Weltwohlfahrtsstaat? (Is There a Global Welfare State?)', in Albert, M. and Stichweh, R. (eds.), *Weltstaat und Weltstaatlichkeit: Beobachtungen globaler politischer Strukturbildungen*. Wiesbaden: VS Verlag für Sozialwissenschaften, pp. 187–208.

Lethbridge, Jane (2004) 'Changing Healthcare Systems in Asia', *Discussion Paper. PSIRU*, London, UK.

Lethbridge, Jane (2005) 'The Promotion of Investment Alliances by the World Bank. Implications for National Health Policy', *Global Social Policy*, 5 (2): 203–225.

Mackintosh, Maureen and Koivusalo, Meri (eds.) (2005) *Commercialization of Health Care. Global and Local Dynamics and Policy Responses*. Basingstoke and New York: Palgrave Macmillan.

Macrae, Joanna, Zwi, Anthony B. and Gilson, Lucy (1996) 'A Triple Burden for Health Sector Reform: "Post"-Conflict Rehabilitation in Uganda', *Social Science Medicine*, 42 (7): 1095–1108.

Mahon, Rianne and McBride, Stephen (eds.) (2008) *The OECD and Global Governance*. Seattle: UBC Press.

Marmot, Michael, Allen, Jessica, Bell, Ruth and Goldblatt, Peter (2012) 'Building of the Global Movement for Health Equity: From Santiago to Rio and Beyond', *The Lancet*, 379 (9811): 181–188.

Martens, Jens (2005) *In Larger Freedom. The Report of the UN Secretary-General for the Millennium+5 Summit 2005*. Berlin: Friedrich Ebert Foundation.

Martens, Kerstin and Jakobi, Anja (eds.) (2010) *Mechanisms of OECD Governance – International Incentives for National Policy Making?* Oxford: Oxford University Press.

Martineau, Tim, Decker, Karola and Bundred, Peter (2004) ' "Brain Drain" of Health Professionals: From Rhetoric to Responsible Action', *Health Policy*, 70 1–10.

McCoy, David (2007) 'The World Bank's New Health Strategy: Reason for Alarm?' *The Lancet*, 369: 1499–1501.

McNeill, Desmond (2005) 'Power and Ideas. Economics and Global Development Policy', in Stone, D. and Maxwell, S. (eds.), *Global Knowledge Networks and International Development*. Oxford, New York: Routledge, pp. 57–71.

Médecins Sans Frontières (2007) *Confronting the Health Worker Crisis to Expand Access to HIV/AIDS Treatment. MSF Experience in Southern Africa*. Johannesburg: Médecins sans Frontières. Available: http://www.msf.org/ source/countries/africa/southafrica/2007/Help_wanted.pdf; (accessed 9 July 2008).

Meseguer, Covadonga (2004) 'What Role for Learning? The Diffusion of Privatisation in OECD and Latin American Countries', *Journal of Public Policy*, 24 (3): 299–325.

Meyer, John W., Boli, John, Thomas, George M. and Ramirez, F. O. (1997) 'World Society and the Nation-State', *American Journal of Sociology*, 103 (1): 144–181.

Mishra, Ramesh (1999) *Globalization and the Welfare State*. Cheltenham: Edward Elgar.

Moran, Michael (1999) *Governing the Health Care State. A Comparative Study of the United Kingdom, the United States and Germany*. Manchester: Manchester University Press.

Moran, Michael (2000) Understanding the Welfare State: The Case of Health Care. *British Journal of Politics and International Relations*, 2: 135–160.

Müller, Katharina (2003) 'The Making of Pension. Privatization in Latin America and Eastern Europe', in Holzmann, R., Orenstein, M. and Rutkowski, M. (eds.), *Pension Reform in Europe: Process and Progress*. Washington, DC: World Bank, pp. 79–110.

Murray, Christopher J. L. and Evans, David B. (eds.) (2003a) *Health Systems Performance Assessment: Debates, Methods and Empiricism*. Geneva: WHO.

Murray, Christopher J. L. and Evans, David B. (2003b) 'Health Systems Performance Assessment: Goals, Framework and Overview', in Murray, C. J. L. and

Evans, D. B. (eds.), *Health Systems Performance Assessment: Debates, Methods and Empiricism*. Geneva: WHO, pp. 3–18.

Musgrove, P. (1999) 'Public Spending on Healthcare: How Are Different Criteria Related', *Health Policy*, 47 (3): 207–223.

Navarro, V. (2001) 'The New Conventional Wisdom: An Evaluation of the WHO Report: Health Systems: Improving Performance', *International Journal of Health Services*, 31 (1): 23–33.

Nelson, Joan M. (2001) 'The Politics of Pension and Health-Care Reforms in Hungary and Poland', in Kornai, J., Haggard, S. and Kaufman, R. R. (eds.), *Reforming the State: Fiscal and Welfare Reform in Post-Socialist Countries*. Cambridge, UK: Cambridge University Press, pp. 235–266.

O'Brien, Robert (2008) 'Global Labour Policy', in Yeates, N. (ed.), *Understanding Global Social Policy*. Bristol: The Policy Press, pp. 123–148.

OECD (1977) *Public Expenditure on Health*. Paris: OECD.

OECD (1987) *Financing and Delivering Health Services. A Comparative Analysis of OECD Countries*. Paris: OECD.

OECD (1992) *The Reform of Health Care. A Comparative Analysis of Seven OECD Countries*. Paris: OECD.

OECD (1993a) OECD *Health Systems. Volume I: Facts and Trends 1960–1991*. Paris: OECD.

OECD (1993b) *Volume II: OECD Health Systems. The Socio-Economic Environment. Statistical References*. Paris: OECD.

OECD (1994) *The Reform of Health Care Systems. A Review of Seventeen OECD Countries*. Paris: OECD.

OECD (1995) *New Directions in Health Policy*. Paris: OECD.

OECD (1996) *Health Care Reform. The Will to Change*. Paris: OECD.

OECD (2000) *A System of Health Accounts*. Paris: OECD.

OECD (2004a) *The OECD Health Project. Private Health Insurance in OECD Countries*. Paris: OECD.

OECD (2004b) *The OECD Health Project. Towards High-Performing Health Systems*. Paris: OECD.

OECD (2005) *The OECD – Organisation for Economic Cooperation and Development*. Paris: OECD.

OECD (2014) *Geographic Variations in Health Care: What Do We Know and What Can Be Done to Improve Health Care System Performance?* Paris: OECD. Available: http://www.keepeek.com/Digital-Asset-Management/oecd/social-issues-migration-health/geographic-variations-in-health-care_9789264216594-en#page4.

OECD and WHO (2006) *OECD Reviews of Health Systems. Switzerland*. Paris: OECD.

Ollila, Eeva and Koivusalo, Meri (2000) 'Values, Ideologies and Evidence-based Recommendations – the World Health Report 2000: WHO's Health Policy Drifting Off Course', in Häkkinen, U. and Ollila, E. (eds.), *The World Health Report 2000. What Does It Tell Us About Health Systems? Analyses from Finnish Experts*. Themes From Finland//2000. Helsinki: National Research and Development Centre for Welfare and Health (Stakes), pp. 3–8.

Ollila, Eeva and Koivusalo, Meri (2002) 'The World Health Report 2000: World Health Organization Health Policy Steering Off Course-Changed Values, Poor Evidence and Lack of Accountability', *International Journal of Health Services*, 32 (3): 503–514.

Olsen, Johan P. (1997) 'European Challenges to the Nation State', in Steunenberg and Vught, F. V. (eds.), *Political Institution and Public Policy*. Dordrecht: Kluwer, pp. 157–188.

Ooms, Gorik, Van Damme, Wim and Temmerman, Marleen (2007) 'Medicines Without Doctors: Why the Global Fund Must Fund Salaries of Health Workers to Expand AIDS Treatment', *PLoS Medicine*, 4 (4): e128.

Or, Zeynep (2002) *Improving the Performance of Health Care Systems: From Measures to Action (a Review of Experiences in Four OECD Countries)*. Paris: OECD.

Orenstein, Mitchell A. (2000) *How Politics and Institutions Affect Pension Reform in Three Postcommunist Countries*. Washington, DC: World Bank.

Orenstein, Mitchell A. (2003) 'Mapping the Diffusion in Pension Innovation', in Holzmann, R., Orenstein, M. A. and Rutkowski, M. (eds.), *Pension Reform in Europe: Process and Progress*. Washington, DC: World Bank, pp. 171–193.

Orenstein, Mitchell A. (2005) 'The New Pension Reform as Global Policy', *Global Social Policy*, 5 (2): 175–202.

Orenstein, Mitchell A. (2008) *Privatizing Pensions. The Transnational Campaign for Social Security Reform*. Princeton, Oxford: Princeton University Press.

Orenstein, Mitchell A. (2011) 'Pension Privatization in Crisis: Death or Rebirth of a Global Policy Trend?' *International Social Security Review,* 64 (3): 65–80.

Ortiz, Isabel (2007) *National Development Strategies Policy Notes Social Policy*. New York: UNDESA.

Peabody, John W. (1995) 'An Organizational Analysis of the World Health Organization: Narrowing the Gap Between Promise and Performance', *Social Science Medicine*, 40 (6): 731–742.

Pollock, A. and Price, D. (2000) 'Rewriting the Regulations: How the WTO Could Accelerate Privatisation in Health Care Systems', *The Lancet*, 356: 1995–2000.

Post, Diahanna L. (2005) 'Standards and Regulatory Capitalism: The Diffusion of Food Safety Standards in Developing Countries', *The Annals of the American Academy of Political and Social Science*, 598: 168–183.

Preker, Alexander S., Scheffler, Richard M. and Bassett, Marc S. (eds.) (2007) *Private Voluntary Health Insurance in Development. Friend or Foe?* Washington, DC: World Bank.

Price, Richard (2003) 'Review Article. Transnational Civil Society and Advocacy in World Politics', *World Politics*, 55: 579–606.

Radelet, Steven (2006) 'The Role of the IMF in Well-Performing Low-Income Countries', in Truman, E. (ed.), *Reforming the IMF in for the 21st Century*. Institute for International Economics, 2006; Center for Global Development Working Paper No. 83. Available at SSRN: http://ssrn.com/abstract =983204Radin.

Reich, Michael R and Takemi, Keizo (2009) 'G8 and Strengthening of Health Systems: Follow-up to the Tokayo Summit', *Lancet*, 373: 508–515.

Roberts, Marc J., Hsiao, William, Berman, Peter and Reich, Michael R. (2008) *Getting Health Reform Right. A Guide to Improving Performance and Equity.* New York: Oxford University Press.

Rockefeller, Foundation (2010) *Catalyzing Change. The System Reform Costs of Universal Health Coverage.* New York: Rockefeller Foundation.

Rothgang, Heinz, Cacace, Mirella, Frisina, Lorraine, Grimmeisen, Simone, Schmid, Achim and Wendt, Claus (2010) *The State and Healthcare. Comparing OECD Countries.* New York: Palgrave Macmillan.

Rothgang, Heinz, Cacace, Mirella, Grimmeisen, Simone and Wendt, Claus (2005) 'The Changing Role of the State in Healthcare Systems', *European Review,* 13 (Supp. No. 1): 187–212.

Ruger, Jennifer Prah (2005) 'The Changing Role of the World Bank in Global Health', *American Journal of Public Health,* 95 (1): 60–70.

Rushton, Simon and William, Owain David (eds.) (2011) *Partnerships and Foundations in Global Health Governance*: Basingstoke: Palgrave Macmillan.

Scheil-Adlung, Xenia (2014) Universal Health Protection: Progress to Date and the Way Forward. Social Protection Policy Papers, Paper 10, Geneva: ILO Social Protection Department. Available: http://apps.who.int/medicinedocs/documents/s21558en/s21558en.pdf.

Seidel, Walter (2003) 'The Report of the Commission on Macroeconomics and Health – A Summary of Findings, Reactions and Follow-Up to the "Sachs-Report" ', in Hein, W. and Kohlmorgen, L. (eds.), *Globalisation, Global Health Governance and National Health Politics in Developing Countries. An Exploration into the Dynamics of Interfaces.* Hamburg: Deutsches Übersee Institute (German Overseas Institute), pp. 117–126.

Sexton, Sarah (2001) 'Trading Health Care Away? GATS, Public Services and Privatisation', *Corner House Briefing,* 23 (June 2001).

Shaw, R. Paul (2007) The Interface Between CSOs and the World Bank; An Input to Global Health or Global Harm? Paper for Discussion. Vancouver, Canada: The Peter Wall Institute for Advanced Study, University of British Columbia.

Siddiqi, J. (1995) *World Health and World Politics: The World Health Organization and the UN System.* London: Hurst and Company.

Simmons, Beth A. and Elkins, Zachary (2004) 'The Globalization of Liberalization: Policy Diffusion in the International Political Economy', *American Political Science Review,* 98 (1): 171–189.

Simmons, Beth A. and Martin, Lisa L. (2002) 'International Organizations and Institutions', in Carlsnaes, W., Kisse, T. and Simmons, B. A. (eds.), *Handbook of International Relations.* Thousand Oaks, CA: Sage, pp. 192–211.

South Centre (2006) *Meeting the Challenges of UN Reform: A South Perspective.* Geneva: Switzerland. Available: http://www.southcentre.org.

St Clair, Asuncion Lera (2006a) 'Global Poverty. The Co-Production of Knowledge and Politics', *Global Social Policy,* 6 (1): 57–77.

St Clair, Asuncion Lera (2006b) 'The World Bank as a Transnational Expertised Institution', *Global Governance,* 12: 77–95.

Stone, Diane (2002) 'Introduction: Global Knowledge and Advocacy Networks', *Global Networks,* 2 (1): 1–11.

Stone, Diane (2003) 'The "Knowledge Bank" and the Global Development Network', *Global Governance,* 9: 43–61.

Stone, Diane and Maxwell, Simon (eds.) (2005) *Global Knowledge Networks and International Development.* Oxford, New York: Routledge.

Stubss, Paul and Wedel, Janine (2015) 'Policy Flexians in Global Order: Contexts, Cases and Consequences', in Kaasch, A. and Martens, K. (eds.), *Actors and Agency in Global Social Governance.* Oxford: Oxford University Press.

Surender, Rebecca and Urbina-Ferretjans, Marian (2015) ' "New Kids on the Block?" The Implications of the BRICS Alliance for Global Social Governance', in Kaasch, A. and Martens, K. (eds.), *Actors and Agency in Global Social Governance.* Oxford: Oxford University Press.

Taipale, Vappu (2000) 'Introduction: There Is a Need for Assessment and Research in Health Policies', in Häkkinen, U. and Ollila, E. (eds.), *The World Health Report 2000. What Does It Tell Us About Health Systems? Analyses from Finnish Experts.* Themes from Finland 7/2000. Helsinki: National Research and Development Centre for Welfare and Health (Stakes). pp. 1–2.

Tarantola, Daniel (2008) 'Global Justice and Human Rights: Health and Human Rights in Practice', *Global Justice: Theory Practice Rhetoric,* 1: 11–26.

Taylor, A. (2002) 'Global Governance, International Health Law and WHO: Looking Towards the Future', *Bulletin of the World Health Organization,* 80 (12): 975–980.

Teegen, Hildy, Doh, Jonathan P. and Vachani, Sushil (2004) 'The Importance of Nongovernmental Organizations (NGOs) in Global Governance and Value Creation: An International Business Research Agenda', *Journal of International Business Studies,* 35: 463–483.

The Global Fund (2012): *The Global Fund Strategy 2012–2016: Investing for Impact.* Geneva: The Global Fund.

Thomas, Carolin and Weber, Martin (2004) 'The Politics of Global Health Governance: Whatever Happened to "Health for All by the Year 2000"?' *Global Governance,* 10: 187–204.

Timmermans, Karin (2004) 'Developing Countries and Trade in Health Services: Which Way Is Forward?' *International Journal of Health Services,* 34 (3): 453–466.

UN (2006) *Delivering as One. Report of the Secretary-General's High-Level Panel on UN System-Wide Coherence.* New York: United Nations.

UN (2014) *The Millennium Development Goals Report.* New York: UN.

UN DESA (1957) *Report on the World Social Situation.* New York: UN.

UN GA (2000) United Nations Millennium Declaration.

UNICEF (2008) *Statement on Toyako Framework on Global Health.* 15 July 2008. New York: UNICEF. Available: http://www.unicef.org/media/media_44776 .html (accessed 3 December 2014).

UN Millennium Project – Task Force On HIV/AIDS, Malaria, TB, and Access to Essential Medicines (2005) *Combating AIDS in the Developing World.* London, Sterling/VA: Earthscan.

Vanduzer, Anthony J. (2005) 'Navigating Between the Poles: Unpacking the Debate on the Implications for Development of GATS Obligations Relating to Health and Education Services', in Petersman, E.-U. (ed.), *Reforming the World Trading System: Legitimacy, Efficiency and Democratic Governance.* Oxford: Oxford, pp. 167–204.

Vaughan, Diane (1999) 'The Dark Side of Organizations: Mistake, Misconduct, and Disaster', *Annual Review of Sociology,* 25 271–305.

Victora, Cesar G., Hanson, Kara, Bryce, Jennifer and Vaughan, J. Patrick (2004) 'Achieving Universal Coverage with Health Interventions', *Lancet,* 364 (1541–48).

Walsh, Julia A. and Warren, Kenneth S. (1980) 'Selective Primary Health Care: An Interim Strategy for Disease Control in Developing Countries', *Social Science and Medicine,* 14C 145–163.

Walt, G. (1994) *Health Policy: An Introduction to Process and Power.* London: Zed Books.

Walt, Gill, Shiffman, Jeremy, Schneider, Helen, Murray, Susan F., Brugha, Ruairí and Gilson, Lucy (2008) ' "Doing" Health Policy Analysis: Methodological and Conceptual Reflections and Challenges', *Health Policy and Planning,* 23 308–317.

Weyland, Kurt (2005) 'Theories of Policy Diffusion. Lessons from Latin American Pension Reform', *World Politics,* 57 262–295.

World Health Assembly (WHA) (1973) Organisational Study on Methods of Promoting the Development of Basic Health Services. *WHA26.35.* WHO.

World Health Assembly (WHA) (1997) Strengthening Health Systems in Developing Countries. *WHA50.27.* WHO.

White, Nigel D. (2002) *The United Nations System: Toward International Justice.* Boulder, CO: Lynne Rienner.

WHO (1998) *Health for All in the 21st Century. A51/5.* Geneva: WHO.

WHO (1999) *The World Health Report 1999. Making a Difference.* Geneva: WHO.

WHO (2000) *The World Health Report 2000: Health Systems: Improving Performance.* Geneva: WHO.

WHO (2005 (updated Reprint) *WHO Framework Convention on Tobacco Control.* Geneva: WHO.

WHO (2006) *Engaging for Health. 11th General Programme of Work, 2006–2015. A Global Health Agenda.* Geneva: WHO.

WHO (2007a) *Everybody's Business. Strengthening Health Systems to Improve Health Outcomes. WHO's Framework for Action.* Geneva: WHO.

WHO (2007b) *The Global Fund Strategic Report to Health System Strengthening. Report from the WHO to the Global Fund Secretariat.* Geneva: WHO. Available: http://www.who.int/healthsystems/GF_strategic_approach_%20HS.pdf.

WHO (2008a) *Statement on the G8 Agreement on Annual Reviews of Progress in Global Health.* Geneva: WHO. Available: http://www.who.int/mediacentre/news/statements/2008/s06/en/ (accessed 3 December 2014).

WHO (2008b) Report on the Expert Consultation on Positive Synergies Between Health Systems and Global Health Initiatives, WHO, Geneva, 29–30 May 2008 WHO: Geneva. Available: http://www.who.int/healthsystems/hs_and_ghi.pdf.

WHO (2008c) World Health Report 2008. Primary Health Care. Now More Than Ever. Geneva: WHO. Available: http://www.who.int/whr/2008/whr08_en.pdf.

WHO (2009a) *Proposed Programme Budget 2010–2011*. Geneva: WHO.

WHO (2009b) *Technical Brief for Policy-Makers. Thinking of Introducing Social Health Insurance? Ten Questions*. Geneva: WHO Department of Health Care Systems Financing.

WHO (2010) *World Health Report 2010: Health Systems Financing: The Path to Universal Coverage*. Geneva: WHO. Available: http://www.who.int/whr/2010/en/.

WHO (2013) *Research for Universal Health Coverage: World Health Report 2013*. Geneva: WHO.

WHO (2014) *Not Merely the Absence of Disease. Twelfth General Programme of Work*. Geneva: WHO.

WHO and World Bank (2013) *Monitoring Progress Towards Universal Health Coverage at Country and Global Levels: A Framework. Joint WHO/World Bank Group Discussion paper, December 2013*. Geneva: WHO. Available: http://www.who.int/healthinfo/country_monitoring_evaluation/UHC_WBG_DiscussionPaper_December 2013.pdf.

WHO and WTO (2002) *WTO Agreements and Public Health: A Joint Guide by the WHO and the WTO Secretariat*. Geneva: WHO/WTO.

WHO CMH (2001) *Macroeconomics and Health: Investing in Health for Economic Development. Report of the Commission on Macroeconomics and Health*. Geneva: WHO.

WHO CSDH (2007) Challenging Inequity Through Health Systems. Final Report Knowledge Network on Health Systems.

WHO CSHD (2008) *Closing the Gap in a Generation. Health Equity Through Action on the Social Determinants of Health. Final Report of the Commission on Social Determinants of Health*. Geneva: WHO.

WHO Europe (1996) *Ljubljana Charter on Reforming Health Care in Europe*. Copenhagen: WHO Regional Office for Europe, available: http://www.euro.who.int/__data/assets/pdf_file/0010/113302/E55363.pdf (accessed 7 December 2014).

WHO Europe (1999) *Health21. The Health for All Policy Framework for the WHO European Region*. Copenhagen: WHO Regional Office for Europe.

WHO Europe (2002) *The European Health Report 2002*. Copenhagen: European Regional Office for Europe.

WHO Europe (2005) *The Health for All Policy Framework for the WHO European Region: 2005 Update*. Copenhagen: WHO Regional Office for Europe.

WHO Europe (2009) *Assessment of Health Care Systems' Crisis Preparedness. Poland*. Copenhagen: WHO Regional Office for Europe. Available: http://www.euro.who.int/__data/assets/pdf_file/0007/112201/E93850.pdf?ua=1.

WHO Europe (2012) *Social Inequalities in Health in Poland*. Copenhagen: WHO Regional Office for Europe. Available: http://www.euro.who.int/__data/assets/pdf_file/0008/177875/E96720.pdf?ua=1.

WHO Europe (2013) *Health 2020. A European Policy Framework and Strategy for the 21st century*. Copenhagen: WHO Regional Office for

Europe. Available: http://www.euro.who.int/__data/assets/pdf_file/0011/ 199532/Health2020-Long.pdf?ua=1.

WHO EB (2013) Universal Health Coverage. Report by the Secretariat. Executive Board 132nd Session, Provisional Agenda Item 10.3. EB132/22. 18 January 2013 available: http://apps.who.int/gb/ebwha/pdf_files/EB132/ B132_22-en.pdf.

WHO/UNICEF (1978) 'Declaration of Alma-Ata'. International Conference on Primary Health Care, 6–12 September 1978 Alma-Ata, USSR.

Wilkinson, Rorden (2002) 'Global Governance. A Preliminary Interrogation', in Wilkinson, R. and Hughes, S. (eds.), *Global Governance. Critical Perspectives*. London/ New York: Routledge, pp. 1–13.

Williams, David and Young, Tom (1994) 'Governance, the World Bank and Liberal Theory', *Political Studies*, 42 (1): 84–100.

Wogart, Jan Peter (2003) 'Global Health Issues and the World Bank's Involvement', in Hein, W. and Kohlmorgen, L. (eds.), *Globalisation, Global Health Governance and National Health Politics in Developing Countries: An Exploration into the Dynamics of Interfaces*. Hamburg: Deutsches Übersee-Institut, pp. 191–202.

Woodward, David (2005) 'The GATS and Trade in Health Services: Implications for Health Care in Developing Countries', *Review of International Political Economy*, 12 (3): 511–534.

World Bank (1980a) *Health Sector Policy Paper*. Washington, DC: World Bank.

World Bank (1980b) *World Development Report 1980*. Washington, DC: World Bank.

World Bank (1987) *Financing Health Services in Developing Countries. An Agenda for Reform*. Washington, DC: World Bank.

World Bank (1992a) Staff Appraisal Report. Poland. Health Services Development Project, available: http://www-wds.worldbank.org/external/default/ WDSContentServer/WDSP/IB/1992/03/27/000009265_3961002053546/ Rendered/PDF/multi0page.pdf, (accessed 7 December 2014).

World Bank (1992b) Poland. Health System Reform. Meeting the Challenge. Report No. 9283-POL, available: http://www-wds.worldbank.org/ external/default/WDSContentServer/WDSP/IB/1992/01/09/000009265_ 3960930055522/Rendered/PDF/multi0page.pdf (accessed 7 December 2014).

World Bank (1993) *World Development Report 1993: Investing in Health*. Oxford, New York et al.: Oxford University Press/ World Bank.

World Bank (1997) *Health, Nutrition, and Population Sector Strategy Paper*. Washington, DC: World Bank.

World Bank (2003) *World Development Report 2004: Making Services Work for Poor People*. Washington, DC: Oxford University Press/World Bank.

World Bank (2007) *Healthy Development. The World Bank Strategy for Health, Nutrition, and Population Results*. Washington, DC: World Bank.

World Bank (2008) Better Outcomes Through Health Reforms in the Russian Federation: The Challenge in 2008 and Beyond. Europe and Central Asia, Human Development Department, Russian Federation Country Management Unit, The World Bank.

World Commission on The Social Dimension of Globalization (2004) *A Fair Globalization: Creating Opportunities for All.* Geneva: ILO.

Yazbeck, Abdo S. (2006) *Economic Viewpoint: Reaching the Poor.* Washington, DC: World Bank.

Yeates, Nicola (2001) *Globalization and Social Policy.* London: SAGE.

Yeates, Nicola (2005) 'The General Agreement on Trade in Services (GATS): What's in It for Social Security?' *International Social Security Review,* 58 (1): 3–22.

Yeates, Nicola (ed.) (2008) *Understanding Global Social Policy.* Bristol: The Policy Press.

Index

Printed and bound by CPI Group (UK) Ltd, Croydon, CR0 4YY